T0209299

YOU ARE WHAT YOU SECRETE

A Practical Guide to Common, Hormone-Related Diseases

Ellis Levin, MD

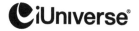

YOU ARE WHAT YOU SECRETE
A PRACTICAL GUIDE TO COMMON,
HORMONE-RELATED DISEASES

iUniverse books may be ordered through booksellers or by contacting:

iUniverse
1663 Liberty Drive
Bloomington, IN 47403
www.iuniverse.com
844-349-9409

Because of the dynamic nature of the Internet, any web addresses or links contained in this book may have changed since publication and may no longer be valid. The views expressed in this work are solely those of the author and do not necessarily reflect the views of the publisher, and the publisher hereby disclaims any responsibility for them.

Any people depicted in stock imagery provided by Getty Images are models, and such images are being used for illustrative purposes only.
Certain stock imagery © Getty Images.

ISBN: 978-1-6632-4252-5 (sc)
ISBN: 978-1-6632-4251-8 (hc)
ISBN: 978-1-6632-4250-1 (e)

Library of Congress Control Number: 2022913130

Print information available on the last page.

iUniverse rev. date: 08/18/2022

INTRODUCTION

A young couple has been desperately attempting to become pregnant. They have tried elaborate maneuvers such as timing their sexual intercourse to a particular day of the month when the woman's morning body temperature is at its peak, determining whether the female makes antibodies to the males sperm, the man wearing boxer rather than jockey shorts, abstaining from sex for periods of time to build up the sperm count, and the female taking antibiotics to cure any vaginal infection. Finally, the couple visits their doctor, disheartened and searching for at least an explanation for their continuing problem. The physician stares thoughtfully out the window for a few minutes, then turns to the couple and announces, "Your problem is hormonal".

However well intentioned, this answer leaves the couple feeling numb and frustrated. After all, what can they possibly do about their hormones? *In fact, what can anyone do*? In this book, we will explore the rational and irrational, the truths and myths of hormone action. The reader will understand that hormone- related diseases can often be treated by changes in life style. Individuals at risk to develop these diseases can be identified by simple screening tests and relatively simple measures can prevent the development or progression of the disease. The reader will understand why the bearded lady and the tiny adult in the circus sideshow share the common problem of abnormal hormone production and action. The contribution of hormones to important health issues will be made clear. For instance, several hormones which are made in the cells of the adrenal glands can cause high blood pressure. The effects of functions of some hormones, like insulin, can often be altered by diet and exercise while severe disease requires drug therapy. The development of breast and prostate cancers are usually dependent on hormone action. In this book, it will be explained that therapy of these diseases is, in part, based on sex hormone manipulations. What is the status of pancreas transplantation, or the artificial pancreas as treatment for diabetes? Is inserting the insulin gene into the body realistic and a potential cure for millions of diabetics? What is the thyroid disease that both the past President and Mrs Bush developed? Is it common and can it be passed among family members? These and many other important questions are answered in this book.

Other hormone related diseases are featured. Osteoporosis is a major disease of the elderly. It is due to accelerated bone loss; and in part the events are caused by insufficient or abnormal hormone action. By detailing the events that result in bone disease, the reader will understand the recommendations on diet, exercise, vitamins, and sex hormone replacement which are offered. Gene replacement therapy or stem cell injections is on the horizon using Crisper-Cas9 technology and will be used widely in the future to correct the abnormality of important genes that code for hormones. These therapies offer the promise of curing diseases of growth and development, fertility, calcium balance, and many other Endocrine (hormone-related) diseases. Providing a missing gene in some forms of cancer will lead to suppression of this deadly disease.

What are these strange substances known as hormones? They are proteins or steroids which are made in almost all body organs, and are then secreted into the blood or body fluid. Proteins are amino acids which have been chemically linked: They provide the basic building material for all tissues. Steroids are made from chemically modified cholesterol and are secreted from the adrenal gland, the ovaries, and the testes. These hormones then travel various distances where they act at target organs in the body to regulate all sorts of important functions. Protein hormones can range in size from several hundred amino acids to only three amino acids. The size of a protein does not determine its' influence. For instance, TRH is only a three amino acid protein hormone. This protein is made in the brain and is crucial for control of thyroid function.

How do hormones act at their target site? Through millions of years of evolution, hormones have become programmed to physically and accurately interact with target organs. The hormone binds a protein called a receptor, which is present on the surface and sometimes interior of the target cell.

This relationship is much like a lock and key. As anyone who has ever tried to open the front door with the back door key knows a specific fit must occur for the door to unlock. After the two proteins bind to each other, a series of chemical events occurs, leading to a unique action for the hormone. For instance, after the protein hormone aldosterone is secreted from the adrenal gland, it travels through the blood to the kidney, where it binds to receptors on the surface of specialized cells in the kidney. The kidney cells regulate salt and water retention in response to aldosterone, resulting in the proper balance of sodium and water throughout the body. If too much aldosterone is secreted, as sometimes occurs from a benign tumor of the adrenal gland, hypertension can result. Therefore, understanding the effects of hormone action provides insight into the disease process, leading to rational treatment recommendations. In this situation, the excess secretion of aldosterone is treated either by removing the adrenal tumor or by prescribing drugs which compete for binding to the aldosterone receptor, antagonizing the effect of the hormone.

As a result of a receptor mainly accepting only one or occasionally two hormones, the body provides a means of dictating that a particular hormone will only affect a particular organ. This selectivity establishes a unique <u>function</u> for that hormone. For instance, it would not be useful for the heart to respond to prolactin, a hormone whose primary purpose is to allow a mother to breast feed milk to her new baby. On the other hand, it is crucial that breast tissue has prolactin receptors that don't bind similar hormones. This is because competition between hormones to bind a receptor could block the action of prolactin.

This issue of hormones acting at receptors made in target cells becomes very important in understanding abnormal hormone action. For instance, there is a particular type of dwarf which occurs in families in the Near East and is named for the physician-investigator who first described these individuals, the Laron Dwarf. These individuals are very short (always less than 5 foot), and disproportionately shaped. Although dwarfing can more commonly result from abnormalities of skeletal development, Laron Dwarfs were originally believed to have decreased production of growth hormone. Growth hormone is the major protein which causes long bone growth at ages 8-15 in older children and adolescents. Strangely, the growth hormone levels of the Laron dwarfs turned out to be quite high, yet these people fail to grow. What has now been appreciated, since the power of molecular biology has been brought to bear on the question, is that they have a mutation (gene abnormality) of the receptor protein. Therefore, the key doesn't fit in the lock, and the individual doesn't grow to full adult height. What is now focused on by much of medical research, is the chemical steps that occur <u>after</u> the hormone binds the receptor, leading to the observed effects of the hormone.

Hormones traditionally have been blamed for causing all kinds of physical and social disorders. As a child, "hormone imbalance" was offered to me as an explanation for why Aunt Rose weighed nearly 300 pounds (never mind the overstocked refrigerator), why Uncle George lost the hair on his head at age 18, and why Cousin Phil is 6' 8" in a family where most of the males could have been jockeys. Dysfunctional hormones were given as an explanation for why Cousin Sue was irritable and tired during "that time of month", why Grandfather Harry was no longer capable of having sexual relations with his wife (only his mistress). Cousin Harriet started having milk discharge from her breasts- only she had never been pregnant! Thus, in any family, many disorders or characteristics can be explained by the effects of hormones, while others are wrongly attributed to these substances. Hormonal action explains why the professional wrestler, Andre the Giant, was 7'6". His tall stature was caused by the excessive secretion of growth hormone from the pituitary gland at the base of the brain, a disorder that occurs usually in teenage years termed "Gigantism". A lack of hormone action also accounts for the curious situation where several well known and well developed Hollywood starlets, are in fact, genetic males!

As I have offered to patients on several occasions, it is one's karma and one's genes that most importantly determine health. In Los Angeles, karma might mean wistfully gazing at the smog-rendered, barely invisible Hollywood sign. Or wishing your lawn snails "a happy day" on your way to the mailbox to pick up the last macrobiotic gardening periodical published north of the planet Neptune. For most people, it means that by understanding the actions of the protein and steroid messengers of the body, one can adopt a life style strategy which leads to better health. At the least, if we understand the basis for disease, we can better accept the afflictions that beset all of us.

Diabetes Mellitus

- What is the disease, **Diabetes Mellitus**?
- Who is at risk to **develop** this devastating illness?
- What can be done to **prevent** the development or complications of Diabetes?
- What are the **newest treatments** for established disease?

J ean Artain nervously relived his past ten days. He couldn't believe that he developed diabetes mellitus at age 16. However three generations of members of his family developed this disease. Doctors where he lives said he should act quickly to minimize the effects of this disease.

At a hospital of the University of California Medical School, his doctors explained they would inject a drug to suppress his immune system, slowing destruction of his pancreas. It seemed to Jean like science fiction, that his own immune system attacks and destroys his pancreas! Why would his cells attack his pancreas?

By injecting him with a drug that inhibits the immune system, the doctors hope to slow the destructive process. Hopefully, his pancreas would recover and resume normal production of the insulin hormone, at least for several years. If suppressing the immune system by taking several different drugs fails, the doctors would then try to transplant a donor human pancreas into his abdomen. Unfortunately, he would still take several drugs to prevent his immune system from rejecting the new pancreas. Alternatively, just pancreas cells that make insulin can be injected into his pancreas to replace the destroyed insulin-producing cells. However, his lymphocytes likely will attack and destroy the cells. Current approaches include surrounding the cells to be injected with material that protects the cells inside the body. These are approaches to cure the disease, but if not completely successful, this treatment could make the diabetes less problematic.

For most diabetics who don't make sufficient insulin to maintain normal glucose levels, these transplant options are not widespread available currently. Therefore injecting short and longer acting insulin and/or taking pills are the usual approaches for treating diabetes. The goal is to prevent poorly controlled diabetes from causing damage to various organs. This includes the eyes, arteries, kidneys, nerves most commonly in the legs, and altered function directly or indirectly in many other organs. When the blood glucose consistently is over 200 mg/dl the excessive glucose causes changes in the proteins in many organs, leading to poor function of the organs mentioned above.

Understanding diabetes causes disease of organs

Unhealthy events from poorly controlled diabetes

In the Unites States, 34 million Americans have diabetes, 90% type 2 Diabetes Mellitus. In early stages, these individuals show resistance to normal insulin action. As a result, the pancreas secretes additional insulin to overcome the insulin resistance in many organs. If the disease progresses and is poorly controlled, insulin production and secretion become very decreased. Also,88 million American adults have prediabetes. Many of the latter individuals will progress to full Diabetes. However there is increased organ dysfunction even in the pre-diabetic state that is increased as glucose control is reduced.

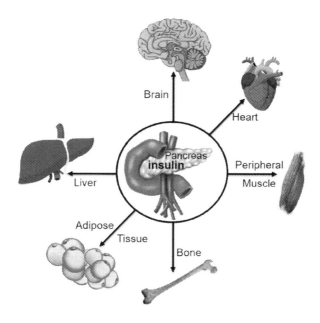

Figure 1-Insulin binds receptors and regulates multiple functions
in numerous organs

Diabetes is more prevalent among non-Hispanic blacks and people
of Hispanic origin than non-Hispanic Asians and non-Hispanic whites.
This parallels obesity in these populations, where the incidence of obesity
in Hispanic and black women is nearly 60% of the populations. Also, men
from these populations are not far behind in being very overweight. In
contrast, Asian men and women are often much less obese.

Medicinal Treatments Background

There is a range of options to treat Diabetes Mellitus. For most individuals,
embracing a regular and moderately strong exercise program is helpful
in getting better control of glucose, Sweating when exercising is very
desirable. Sweating shows that stored fat in the body is being used for
energy that is important for exercising.

Exercising along with eating a healthy diet is very important. For overweight or obese individuals, decreasing the food portions, carbohydrates (like bread), and fat that one eats at meals. The two diets strongly suggested for good health overall and helpful for diabetics are the Dash diet and the Mediterranean diet. These diets can be found online from one's computer looking at recommendations from the American Diabetes Association and the American Nutrition Society.

Excessive weight leads to the resistance of insulin action in most organs of the body. Insulin resistance as mentioned is very common in the early stages of Type 2 Diabetes that often occurs mostly in adults. Children or young adults are more likely to develop Type 1 Diabetes, All diabetics show some resistance to the normal functions of insulin.

Importantly, insulin stimulates the uptake of the sugars, glucose or fructose (converted to glucose), from what we ingest. Glucose is changed into a fat, triglycerides, and often stored in our fat cells (adipocytes). This is used for energy when exercising, or when someone skips a meal or during sleep. Importantly, because of insulin resistance, the triglyceride fat is stored in other cells. As a result, the fat is taken up by the liver. This causes fatty liver disease that can progress to liver failure and/or liver cancer in some individuals. Also, the fat is taken up by cells in the lining of blood vessels. This contributes to the development of atherosclerosis. This process can result in blood clots of large arteries, generating strokes and heart attacks (myocardial infarction). The latter is especially likely when glucose is poorly controlled and cholesterol and triglycerides are very high in blood and organs.

To further elaborate, newly diagnosed type 1 diabetes (also known as insulin-requiring diabetes) is often treated with medicines to suppress the immune system to prevent or delay full disease onset by years. Diabetes occurs when the major immune cell, the lymphocyte, attacks and destroys its target, in this case the insulin-secreting cells in the pancreas. Normally, the lymphocyte targets viruses, bacteria, and other infectious agents, or foreign particles or proteins which are inhaled. A normally functioning immune system is essential to live a long and healthy life. For unexplained reasons, the immune system no longer recognizes the pancreas as being a part of the body, and specifically attacks the insulin producing beta cells, while sparing other cells that make up the pancreas. Several proteins found in the pancreas have been identified as proteins targeted by the immune system. Preventing the immune cell causing destruction of the endocrine pancreas at an early stage, diabetes can be prevented or significantly delayed. Further explanation can be found at the American Diabetes Society website, and the website of the Endocrine Societies of England and the USA.

Diabetes- who is at risk?

What defines a risk to develop this disease? This is important because Diabetes is a major contributor to blindness, heart attack, loss of limbs, kidney failure, and premature death? To answer these questions, we should understand how the body normally uses glucose, in the blood.

Glucose is a fuel that is essential for normal function of most cells in the body. Glucose comes from the food and beverages we consume or is produced in the liver and is then secreted into the blood. Insulin secretion is carefully regulated by the body, increasing as much as 1,000% in response to a meal, compared to between meal secretion. The secreted insulin's first action is to bind to specific protein receptors in the liver to shut off new glucose production. After this, insulin travels throughout the body in the blood, and causes glucose and amino acid uptake by muscle and fat cells. The cells then use the glucose for energy and the amino acids to make new proteins, essential for the health and function of the body.

Type 1 diabetes results when the body can no longer make sufficient insulin.

Diabetes mellitus is diagnosed when an individual has fasting blood glucoses higher than 110 miligrams/dl, on two separate occasions, or 150, 2 hours after a meal. One test that is routinely measured to give a more overall measurement of glucose control is hemoglobin A1c (HgbA1c) in the blood. Another is fructosamine that can tell the effects of new or changed medicines on serum glucose within 2 weeks. If a person has typical symptoms of diabetes, the glucose is often over 200 and the diagnosis is made. These symptoms might include excessive drinking, urinating or hunger, weakness, or blurred vision.

Keto-acidosis

Severely affected individuals can be extremely ill. These people will come to a hospital emergency room with nausea, vomiting, and abdominal pain, dehydration, and extreme tiredness, or even coma. So profound may be the consequences when this disease surfaces that an individual's blood may be acidic (like acid), leading to depressed heart and lung function, abnormal heart rhythm (arrythmias) and death if not treated. When insulin production by the pancreas is very low, then glucose in the blood can not be taken up by many cells that use glucose as a source of energy. To make up for this, in the liver, cells break down fat into ketones but this can result in too much ketones that cause the blood to be like acid. That is why these people are given insulin dripped into veins, often in the intensive care unit of the hospital, and this occurs until better control of glucose and decreased ketones and acidic blood results.

Therefore, we must try to identify people at excessive risk, and either prevent the disease, or at least identify diabetes in its early stages. By early identification, combination of changes in life-style and appropriate therapy can strongly prevent most of the unwanted effects of high glucose throughout the body. It is important to identify and intervene early on to prevent damage that can't be reversed. For instance, if early stages of neuropathy (numbness and tingling, progressing to pain of nerves most often in the legs) can be identified and treated by excellent glucose control, the nerve damage can be repaired by the body and not progress further.

Altered genes and diabetes

Unfortunately, we have only begun to understand the genetics of diabetes, abnormal genes that promote the development of this disease. We know, for instance, that the risk of developing diabetes is significantly increased if a first degree relative has this disease. This is true for Type 1 Diabetes but even more so for Type 2 Diabetes. We know that certain patterns of chromosomal and gene expression predispose people to this disease. For instance, there is a part of chromosome 6 where several genes determine one's immune function. If an abnormality of this region exists in a person, their chances of developing diabetes increases as much as 20 fold. A group of doctors in Boston published studies showing that an abnormality of these genes on chromosome 6 alters proper communication between cells of the immune system. This lack of communication is predicted to lead to the immunity cells attacking normal cells in the pancreas organ, exactly the situation in type I diabetes.

Complications of Diabetes

General Prevention Strategies

Life Style Intervention

Several strategies should be employed. First, diet is important. Every diabetic knows that he or she must generally avoid excessive sugar, to keep the blood glucose from rising too high. Instead, the American Diabetic

Association recommends that 30% of calories should come from *complex* carbohydrates, not simple sugars that are carbohydrates. Carbohydrates should contain high fiber, vitamins, and minerals and be low in sugar, fat, and salt. Potatoes should be avoided if overweight, and rather rice or wheat grains are preferred. Approximately 30% of calories should come from low fat protein including fish or chicken, or lean meat. Another 30% of calories should be from fat. The fat should be mono-unsaturated or even better, *polyunsaturated fat* and trans-fat should be avoided. Polyunsaturated fat raises HDL (high density lipoprotein, the good form of cholesterol), and improves control of blood glucose. Fish, walnuts, and soy are examples of food high in polyunsaturated fat. Mono-unsaturated fat should be provided by cooking with olive oil, an essential part of the Mediterranean diet. Look up the further details of healthy diets on-line from the American Society for Nutrition.

Simple sugars such as glucose and fructose that are seen in most foods should be very limited. Importantly, fructose is directly converted to triglyceride fat and stored in the liver, promoting the fatty liver syndrome. Thus, diabetics should only occasionally eat modest amounts of sweets, as part of their meals. Excessive sugar leads to weight increases, more insulin resistance, and worsening control of blood glucose. Therefore, diabetics should limit high sugar desserts. In pre-diabetics, intermittent fasting would enable weight loss and enhanced action of the insulin their pancreas produces and secretes. The intermittent fasting (total calories of 400-500 calories for the entire day) should occur two days a week. In pre-diabetes, many universities have published that replacing starches with more mono-unsaturated fat (cook with olive oil) reduces triglyceride levels in the blood,

It has been reported that diets high in fiber delay absorption of food in the intestine. This results in a more gradual challenge to the body. This smooths out the surge of calories which overwhelms the limited ability of the pancreas to increase insulin secretion in Type 2 Diabetics. High fiber diet also reduces the amount of insulin needed to be injected in

Type 1 Diabetics. Smaller amounts of food also lead to increased action of injected insulin. Increased fiber is gained from bran, vegetables, and non-absorbable starches. Increased fiber in the diet is convincingly linked to preventing development of cancer of the colon and heart disease, in both non-diabetics and diabetics. Thus, this dietary strategy is of benefit to all family members.

If overweight, a 5% weight loss provides some benefits, but up to 15% weight loss leads to optimal prevention of the complications of diabetes, due in part to better glucose control. There are some medications, such as Qsymia that can often result in an average 10% weight loss over 1 year that is maintained by diet and exercise. In very obese individuals, bariatric surgery by an experienced surgeon should be considered.

Additionally, the diabetic should ideally eat smaller meals per day. This prevents overwhelming the bodies' limited ability to make insulin by presenting smaller amounts of food (and sugar) to be processed. This is very applicable to Type 2 Diabetics. Smaller meals decreases the need for large amounts of insulin to control the blood glucose. Injecting smaller amounts of insulin is important. Many studies indicate that large amounts of insulin by itself accelerate the development of blood vessel diseases, like atherosclerosis. Atherosclerosis results in heart disease and is a major cause of death in the diabetic. Studies show that insulin in high concentrations stimulates production and secretion of a hormone which is made in the cells lining blood vessels. This hormone, called Endothelin, has been proposed to play a role in the development of atherosclerosis. This contributes to damage to the heart, resulting from a heart attack (myocardial infarction). This is but one way that excessive insulin can accelerate vascular disease, In addition insulin promotes excessive production of triglycerides, a fat that contributes to the development of atherosclerosis. New strategies to reduce excessive insulin production and enhance insulin action in Type 2 Diabetes is important and can be a result of diet and exercise. Thus lifestyle changes can also help lower the high amounts of insulin needed in Type 1 Diabetics. These strategies help prevent stroke or heart attack. Several forms of cancer development are also enhanced by excessive insulin secretion. This is especially important for breast cancer in women and colon cancer in men and women.

But what happens if a diabetic needs large amounts of insulin to adequately control the blood glucose? Our goal in controlling diabetes is to keep all blood glucoses under 200 mg. This is the catch 22 of diabetic therapy- it is therefore very important to control blood glucose even if requiring injecting large amounts of insulin. Glucose under 200 is also the goal of life-style changes if possible, as non-medicine-based strategies.

A typical daily diet which includes needed amounts of fiber and which provides 2,000 calories is illustrated in table 1. If the individual is overweight the recommended portion size should be reduced in half.

Table 1- Recommended Diabetic Daily Diet (2,000 calories)	
Breakfast	Bran Flakes (1 cup) Banana (1/2) 1% Milk (1 cup)
Lunch	Chicken Sandwich (1/4 pound) with tomato pear
PM Snack	Whole Grain Toast (2 pieces) Orange
Dinner	Lean Steak (3 ounces) Brown Rice (1 cup) with margarine Broccoli (1/2 cup) Strawberries (1 1/4 cup)
Bedtime Snack	Popcorn, air popped (3 cups), and 1% milk (1 cup)
Snacks not needed for all diabetics	

This diet provides the 2,000 calories as 55% carbohydrate, 15% protein and 30% as fat. It also provides 40 grams of fiber, the recommended amount for daily consumption. The need for weight loss should reduce the calories to 1000-1200 per day and less non-fiber carbohydrates such as limiting bread. Speaking to a nutritionist/dietician should be important in planning a menu that fits your needs.

Diet sodas can be consumed in moderation and should be replaced when possible by drinking water and "mineral water" that is usually safe, unless added salt or sugar is apparent. Coffee and tea by themselves do not contain significant calories. A can of beer contains a lot of calories and should be consumed in place of fat (such as an exchange for a serving of salad dressing), perhaps three-four times a week at most if desired. Detailed diet information as mentioned can be obtained from the American Diabetes Association and also from the American Nutrition Society.

Another strategy to prevent or lessen the need for diabetic treatment is exercise. The body utilizes calories much more effectively when regular exercise is part of one's daily activities. This results, in part, because insulin acts much more effectively to promote glucose entry into cells during exercising rather than resting muscle and fat cells. Exercising muscle demands glucose (or calories) as a fuel: By increasing the uptake of calories into muscle, the blood glucose is lowered. In addition, physical training is associated with lower insulin levels. It has been observed in many diabetic patients that their insulin requirements fall markedly during periods of regular, moderate exercise. Long term, these effects could also prevent or lessen the complications of diabetes. This strategy is equally effective in the diabetic who requires insulin or pill therapy. Increased physical activity *prevents the development of type II diabetes*, especially in high-risk individuals.

What constitutes a good exercise program? A typical routine that is sufficient for achieving good cardiovascular tone, and utilization of calories, would be to swim a third of a mile, 3-4 times per week. An equivalent program would be to strenuously walk on flat surfaces for 4 miles, 3-4 times per week. Bicycling 6-8 miles, 3-4 times per week is also recommended. Jogging or moderate to high impact aerobics damages joints like the ankles. The previously mentioned programs of exercise are less traumatic and equally beneficial, as preferred. It is important that the exercise results in sweating. Sweating is an indication that cells are burning stored fat (oxidation) for energy while exercising. This is critical to reduce weight and enhance insulin action, thus reducing the amount of insulin secreted or injected.

Complications of Diabetes

Eye Disease

When high blood and tissue levels of glucose persist over many years, important changes occur. In the eye, this means that the lens processes glucose abnormally. This leads to swelling of the lens, blurred vision, and cataract formation, well known complications of Diabetes. In the interior of the eye of the diabetic, the retina grows new blood vessels which can pull and may eventually tear the retina, the deep layer of our eyes. Also, the new blood vessels can lead to bleeding or swelling of the interior of the eye. These events result in decreased vision, or even blindness. Thus, if we can prevent the high levels and abnormal processing of glucose, we can often prevent these complications of diabetes.

In one study from England, one thousand diabetic patients were examined. Approximately 10 percent had severe-vision threatening eye disease, requiring immediate treatment. Diabetics also have an increased rate of glaucoma. Another eye complication resulting from diabetes is the deposit of protein material in the eye, called hard or soft exudates. Exudates by themselves do not represent a threat to vision.

Accelerated blood vessel thickening and leaking can cause the bleeding in the eye. This is a worrisome complication of diabetes. Most feared are new blood vessel formation on the retina or central part of the interior of the eye, the disc. These blood vessels arise because thickening of the eye arteries leads to decreased blood flow, These results cause poor blood supply and decreased oxygen. Although new blood vessels formed to increase the oxygen level. Unfortunately, the new vessels pull on the retina, resulting in tearing and detachment. Also, these fragile blood vessels are prone to bleeding, destroying vital structures in the eye. At present, laser therapy is the recommended treatment, to seal these vessels and stop their growth. This prevents retinal detachment or large hemorrhage in the eye.

Preventing the eye complications of Diabetes involves tightly controlling blood glucose and starting early laser therapy for proliferative eye disease before permanent damage occurs. Hypertensive (high blood pressure) diabetics have a much greater rate of eye complications. This risk is decreased with good control of blood pressure. A careful study from England in Diabetics with eye disease have shown that excellent control of Diabetes for 2-3 years does not reverse their eye disease. However, progression of the eye disease may be stopped. A better understanding of the gene background may be helpful. This information could provide an answer to the question, why do some individuals develop these complications, while other diabetics with comparable blood glucose do not develop eye disease. This information will allow us to practice preventive medicine and avoid these devastating problems in the future.

Table 2- Abnormalities of the eye in Diabetes	
Cataracts	
Glaucoma	
	Hemorrhage
	Exudates
	Retinal Detachment
	New Blood Vessel Formation
	Neuropathy

Diabetics can develop severe *abnormalities of the nervous system*. They may develop numbness or tingling in the nerves of their arms and legs. There can be pain that develops and disrupts sleep. These symptoms often follow the loss of the ability to detect vibration or position. These abnormalities result from function disruption and death of the nerves that come out of the spinal cord and provide sensation to the arms and legs. This condition occurs from chronic elevations of glucose above 200 mg, With time, sensation over many parts of the body is lost.

At present, we can't strongly predict with great accuracy who will or won't develop nerve problems. However *poor glucose control always is involved*. Therefore, we want to prevent this outcome of Diabetes. If we control the Diabetes/blood glucose early we can often prevent progression of the nerve damage.

As a result of loss of feeling in the feet, diabetics may injure themselves without realizing it. Often, diabetics will be found to have ulcers or cuts of the feet which they didn't know they had developed. More than once, I have found pins or needles in the feet of diabetics who lack sensation, discovered after careful examination or x-rays of the feet. It is important that individuals who develop this complication should not walk without shoes, to prevent injury. Also, well-fitting shoes will prevent skin breakdown, ulcers, and infections, which can lead to amputation of the feet. Diabetics should regularly check between their toes for fungal infections and ulcers or cuts. The latter provide an entrance for bacteria, causing bacterial infection. Individuals with elevated blood glucose have a much higher rate of developing certain infectious diseases, including tuberculosis and fungal infections. Diabetic women have a higher rate of urine infections than non-diabetic women. More important, they have greater difficulty in fighting infections, because their immune cells do not function normally.

Diabetics may also develop a second nerve disorder. This disorder most often presents as severe pain and weakness of a single extremity, most often a leg. Fortunately, it usually resolves over several months, and therefore only requires pain medicines as needed for treatment.

Prevention

What can be done to prevent the development of nerve diseases? Nerve complications of Diabetes occurs in response to abnormal processing of glucose when blood glucose exceeds 200mg. Therefore, it is important to tightly control blood glucose as the main preventive strategy. This can be accomplished as already detailed, by a combination of diet, exercising, and medications, as needed. Several human trials have tried to restore the nerve levels of a sugar called myo-inositol, hoping this would prevent or stabilize neuropathy. This attempt has not been successful, nor does the vitamin thiamine prevent neuropathy: Thus, *good control of blood glucose and care of feet and legs* remains the best strategy to prevent these complications.

The difficulty is that there is no indicator as to which diabetics are particularly predisposed to this complication, and thus would benefit by early therapy, Hopefully, genetic analysis will provide us with the insight regarding this question in the future.

Treatment

Once symptoms of neuropathy develop, the diabetic has several choices. Pain medications can reduce the pain suffering. Pregabalin (Lyrica) or Gabapentin (Neurontin) are each often used as first line drugs to reduce pain. Anti-depressants like elavil are best used at night to help Diabetics fall asleep with minimal pain. Tegretol, is useful in some diabetics with painful neuropathy that did not respond to the mentioned drugs. A doctors' help is needed to monitor rare but important side effects of Tegretol. Another treatment is a cream which the diabetic can rub onto the painful area. This cream, capsaicin, contains ground up chili peppers. The peppers contain a natural chemical which opposes the action of a hormone called substance P, implicated in the pain due to nerve disorders. The starting amount needed of these drugs is often different for individuals, based in part as to how advanced Diabetes and nerve damage has progressed.

Kidney

Another organ that may be severely affected by long term Diabetes is the kidney. It is estimated that approximately 40 % of type 1 diabetics will develop significantly impaired kidney function, and kidney failure. Kidney failure requires dialysis, often after 20 years of diabetes. After seven years of progressing kidney (renal) failure, 50% of diabetics will have died unless kidney transplantation occurs. Thus, preventing the development and progression of kidney disease due to Diabetes is a major public health goal in our country. Diabetes and the abnormal function of the kidney may result from significant loss of protein from the body, and abnormal handling of salt, water, and potassium. Although many diabetics develop significant kidney disease, others have relatively normal renal function. *What distinguishes the two groups is unknown*, but it is probably related to several genes which are inherited from one's parents. The presence of the protein albumin in the urine predicts who will develop diabetic kidney disease. This is a marker to intervene with medication that limits disease progression of this organ.

The best preventive strategy of avoiding this complication is to tightly control the blood glucose, using whatever combination of treatments is effective to achieve this aim. Many diabetics also develop hypertension, and the combination of poorly controlled diabetes and high blood pressure is lethal to the kidney. Thus, a combination of salt restriction, weight reduction and medicines to control high blood pressure, coupled with glucose control is essential to maintain relatively normal kidney function. Recently, it has been suggested that restricting dietary protein and phosphorous in the diet retards the development of renal failure. More studies are needed to confirm this potential preventive strategy, but this idea can be used in some patients, under supervision of a physician. To summarize, the diabetic individual who develops severe renal disease may require dialysis and possible transplantation, options which should serve to inspire diabetics to actively control their disease in the early stages.

Impotence

A complication which male diabetics may develop is impotence. The basis for this complication is not completely understood. It probably results from a combination of nerve damage and decreased blood supply to the penis, often due to accelerated arteriosclerosis. As found by a team of Boston University researchers, male diabetics lack the ability to relax the smooth muscle of the penis. This has the effect that blood cannot enter and swell the shaft of the penis. The normal process might be visualized as water rushing into a dry lake bed when the flood gates of a dam are opened, on a much smaller scale. The lack of smooth muscle relaxation prevents swelling of the penis with blood, which is necessary for a normal erection. The reason for lack of relaxation is mainly a deficiency of a gas, nitric oxide, made in blood vessel cells.

Yes, a gas, nitric oxide. This gas is created when the amino acid, arginine, which is present in many foods, is converted into nitric oxide by cells that line the blood vessels. Nitric oxide is a potent dilator (relaxing) substance. Lack of production of nitric oxide in large arteries has been strongly implicated in developing arteriosclerosis, and probably contributes to the death of heart cells after a heart attack. Why diabetics can't produce sufficient nitric oxide is not known. It may be related to damage of the lining of blood vessels, associated with high blood glucose. This knowledge provides a basis for treatment of this complication. A strategy presumes that the cells are still capable of making nitric oxide in sufficient amounts. Controlling diabetes to lessen the nerve or blood vessel damage is still the soundest preventive strategy. Medical treatment has often used Silendafil, also known as Viagra, that increases cell production of nitric oxide. This causes artery dilation and the flow of blood into the penis producing erect and rigid state.

One other factor must be considered. In evaluating impotence in a diabetic, the blood levels of the male sex hormone, testosterone, must be measured to rule out possible deficiency. This should be *done in the early morning.* If testosterone levels are low, every two weeks injection of testosterone or daily testosterone patches will help restore potency but the blood flow is the most important contributor.

If these strategies fail, impotence can be treated either with penile implants or suction devices. Penile implants require the insertion of a rubber or silastic rod into the penis, with a small pump that can be inflated when a man desires an erection. This device gives new meaning to the phrase "pump it up". The procedure is costly, and has, in my opinion, too many potential complications. A good alternative is the suction devices which are currently available. These devices can provide an erection which can last for up to an hour. Basically, the male places the cylinder-shaped structure over the shaft of the penis, and a rubber ring constricts the penis at the base. He then inflates the device, producing a vacuum which draws blood into the penis. The blood is prevented from leaving the penis by the rubber constricting ring. The cylinder is then removed, and the erection is maintained. Once a male wants to relieve the constriction, and lose his erection, he simply removes the rubber ring. This apparatus has proven very successful and desirable by many male diabetics who desire sexual relations despite being impotent. This device is equally successful in the treatment of impotence in non-diabetics.

Accelerated Vascular Disease

Another severe complication that diabetics develop is accelerated blood vessel disease of arteries, due to arteriosclerosis. The causes of the accelerated blood vessel disease are several. Diabetics often have very high levels of the fat called triglyceride, and increased low density lipoprotein cholesterol (LDL-cholesterol), in their blood. They also have low HDL cholesterol; When abundant, HDL cholesterol is associated with lower heart attacks. The reason for these developments is that the fat producing proteins are normally regulated in part by insulin, which is often lacking in the type 1 diabetic. Also, the platelets of diabetics function abnormally and are more likely to form a clot inside blood vessels.

Diabetics also often have hypertension, creating a double whammy for the blood vessel. It is felt that high blood glucose can accelerate the aging process of the blood vessel, making it less flexible and predisposing to thrombus (clot) formation. Achieving prevention of accelerated vascular disease begins with the previously suggested strategies for preventing other complications of diabetes. In addition, all other factors, such as elevated blood pressure and excessive triglyceride or LDL cholesterol, should be rigorously controlled. Finally, a baby aspirin each day can significantly decrease the rate of heart attack or stroke in all men over 45 years of age; the diabetic is no exception to this recommendation. After the age of 70, the aspirin daily use should be stopped because of increased bleeding that can occur.

A new understanding of how excessive glucose can contribute to several complications of diabetes has been proposed by Dr Anthony Cerami and his colleagues. They proposed that high blood glucose leads to stiffening of the elastic and collagen fibers of many tissues, due to changes in the chemistry of these tissues. This can lead to blood vessel disease. This same phenomenon contributes to other changes of aging, including stiffness and lack of flexibility and arthritis.

Miscellaneous Complications

Diabetics often have abnormalities of the stomach and intestines. The decreased function of the stomach leads to failure of food to move into the intestines. This can lead to bloating, nausea and vomiting. Also, because food is irregularly passed to the intestine, absorption is not regular. When a diabetic takes insulin, poor absorption of food can lead to severe hypoglycemia (low blood glucose). Often, diabetics will benefit from the drug metoclopramide, which improves function of the stomach. The antibiotic erythromycin also can improve this function of the stomach.

Diabetics can develop diarrhea. Contributing factors include bacterial growth and poor contracting function in the intestines but other causes are not known. Use of anti-diarrheal, over-the counter drugs such as Lomotil, and control of blood glucose helps. Unfortunately, our knowledge about this complication is incomplete.

Treatment of Established Type 1 Diabetes Mellitus

To this point, I have discussed a program to avoid or delay the early and later development of diabetes. However, many individuals already have this disease and look forward to new definitive therapies and treatments. As expected, diet and exercise have important roles in managing established diabetes, as part of an overall treatment plan. This section will review current and future therapies, including pill or insulin treatment, immunotherapy, the artificial pancreas, insulin pump treatment, pancreas transplantation, and the brightest hope for the future, gene therapy.

Insulin

The most important therapy for the type 1 diabetic is insulin replacement. This treatment is necessary because most type 1 diabetics have lost the ability to make sufficient insulin in their pancreas. Insulin is usually given by injection just below the skin. The problem is that this avoids a first important action of insulin that occurs from insulin secreted from the pancreas. That is, insulin injected under the skin does not first reach the liver to stop glucose production in this organ. There are also other functions of insulin in the liver which are not well understood. However, these liver effects from insulin made in the pancreas are important but are bypassed by insulin injection under the skin. From attempts to administer insulin by nasal spray or inhalation or swallowing insulin pills, each has difficulties for replacing injected insulin.

There have been attempts to give insulin in pill or capsule form. This method results in insulin effects somewhat similar to action of insulin secreted from the pancreas. Unfortunately, breakdown of insulin by acid and digestive chemicals in the stomach prevents this method of treatment form being useful. However, in the future, pharmaceutical companies may put insulin into a capsule which prevents insulin destruction. The goal is for good absorption in the intestine. An additional benefit of oral insulin is cost savings, since needles, syringes, and alcohol swabs would be unnecessary

Currently, technology-engineered human insulin has replaced animal insulin. The insulins used today are produced in bacteria, and cause less allergic reactions, because they are pure insulin with little contaminating protein. As a result, less skin reactions occur at the site of injection. The current goal of insulin treatment is making the blood glucose levels similar to a non-diabetic, in order to prevent complications of this disease. Injecting the smallest amount of insulin possible to provide good control of blood glucose is a goal. Large nationwide studies involving several University Hospitals determined that having a hemoglobinA1c of 7.0% produces very significant reductions in the complications of diabetes. This is compared to poorly controlled diabetics. In older men and women, such as 70-80 years, it is acceptable to settle for a hemoglobinA1c of 7.5 or even 8.0

Studies aiming for even stronger reduction of the HgbA1c in most humans (to 6.5 or lower) has not shown a further reduction in complications, and one large study showed increased death. Very tight control however does seem to benefit younger diabetics who are likely to develop complications after 10-15 years of having this disease.

Another common method of giving insulin is through an insulin pump, usually attached to a needle which lies just under the skin. The insulin pump, which is often hooked to a belt, provides a steady insulin infusion, and can be programmed for injecting bursts of insulin prior to meals. Now continuous glucose monitors can be linked to and control the injection rate of insulin from the pump, based on sampling of blood glucose multiple times. This method has been successful in many diabetics to eliminate high levels of glucose or low glucose, resulting in spending most time in the desired glucose range of 90-150.

Insulin and pill treatment

In some type 1 diabetics, treatment with the combination of pills and insulin is desirable. Approximately 15% of overweight, older diabetics can initially benefit from combined treatment, gaining better control of their blood glucose. Combination therapy, along with lifestyle changes, results in better control of blood glucose and lowers the overall amount of insulin that is injected to achieve glucose goals. Newer drugs will be discussed in depth in the section on Type 2 Diabetes treatment.

Once therapy is started, it is important for the diabetic to determine blood glucose levels and change the insulin regimen as situations change. For instance, if a diabetic knows that he/she will exercise heavily on a certain day, the insulin amount should be cut back by 25-35%. Also, if a diabetic becomes ill, and can't take in food because of vomiting or feeling poorly in general, they should decrease their total insulin by 50%. It is important that diabetics do not completely stop their insulin even if they are not eating! This is because the *stress of the illness, like an infection, can cause the release of hormones that increase blood glucose.*

One of the most common situations which results in the hospitalization of the diabetic occurs when the individual stops insulin during an illness because they weren't eating. Diabetics should measure their glucose levels using a home glucometer once or twice a day and make appropriate adjustments. As mentioned, continuous glucose monitors (CGM) have become available for diabetics to have a better understanding of their glucose control. A good indicator of overall glucose control is the glycosylated hemoglobin (HgA1c). This modification of hemoglobin reflects blood glucose levels during the previous six weeks, a good overall assessment of the success in controlling glucose tightly.

Future Therapy for Diabetes Mellitus

Two new methods of restoring the body's ability to make insulin will be used in the future. Currently, a limited number of diabetics are undergoing pancreas transplantation especially at University Hospitals, such as in Minnesota and Florida. These individuals receive a donor pancreas, often together with kidney transplant if needed. Another method is to isolate the insulin producing region of the pancreas, place it in a capsule, and inject these cells into the abdomen. The results from patients who have undergone pancreas transplantation is encouraging but is limited by availability of a donor pancreas. The resulting control of blood glucose appears to be very similar to control *in normal, non-diabetics*. The complications of this procedure are mainly related to the drugs that prevent the body from rejecting the transplanted pancreas. However, short term results do not indicate this problem to be severe. However, a long term (such as 15 years) experience is not known. The limitations of this technology applied to the millions of type 1 diabetics worldwide is the cost and lack of enough pancreas donors.

One therapy of choice for the future will be gene (DNA) replacement. This technique is already being used to potentially cure other diseases that are due to an abnormality of a single gene. For Diabetes, the gene which produces insulin could be placed into cells of the pancreas which have not been damaged, or into other cells lining the abdomen. It has been shown in rats, that the insulin gene is taken up by cells, which then leads to the production of insulin.

Several major problems need to be overcome, before this therapy can be offered to diabetics. First, it would be best if the gene was only expressed in cells of the pancreas or abdominal lining. Therefore, techniques must be developed to selectively express this gene. Second, regulation of blood glucose is the result of balance between several hormone systems that regulate insulin production. Regulation of the insulin gene placed into cells from a diabetic rat, often does not show the same control of insulin secretion as *normal* rats or humans. These problems however, are not insurmountable and it is likely that insulin gene therapy can be a treatment in the near future.

A second treatment on the horizon is using islet cells from the pig, placed by small incision into the abdomen of humans. The pig islets produce pork insulin, which is well tolerated by humans, and can establish its own blood supply and be regulated similarly to the normal human pancreas. A huge technical problem with this approach is that the human body recognizes the pig islet cells as foreign, stimulating a violent rejection process. This is a problem but could be overcome by administering drugs to suppress this reaction, comparable to what is done for heart, liver, or kidney transplants.

However, it has recently found that the islets can be placed into protective capsules that allow the secreted insulin to get out into the body. Importantly, the capsules don't let immune cells into the capsules and therefore protect the islet cells. As a result, the encapsulated islets are tolerated by the human body and are not rejected. This approach holds great promise. Large numbers of islets are needed to cure the 1 million Type 1 diabetics in the United States but that will require using pig islets. If nothing else, interest in this approach will benefit those who invest in pork belly futures on the Chicago Mercantile stock market. A silver lining.

Type 2(II) Diabetes

A second form of this disease occurs generally in the middle aged or elderly individual. There is a maturity onset of Diabetes in youth (MODY) but this is not common and can often be treated with sulfonylurea drugs like Glimeperide These diabetics are often very overweight, and do not initially lack insulin production, *but are resistant to the effects of their own insulin*. This form of Diabetes in early stages is called Type II or non-insulin dependent diabetes. This type of diabetes accounts for ~90% of the disease, or 31 million Americans. It is estimated that as many as 43% of first-degree relatives of Type II Diabetics will develop this disease. Also as many as 96 million Americans are pre-diabetic and as many as 10% become diabetic each year. The earlier these individuals begin a healthy lifestyle and perhaps take the drug metformin is a successful way to prevent progression to the disease, Diabetes.

Research into the cause of Type 2 Diabetes has found that these individuals have both decreased insulin receptor numbers and abnormal receptor functioning. As a result, the ability of insulin to promote the uptake of blood glucose into cells is decreased. This is insulin resistance. Also this disease is in part due to the altered production or state of proteins which normally help insulin accomplish its important functions.

The type 2 diabetic often has fewer complications than the type 1 diabetic; but still can develop similar problems at a lower rate. Severe complications in Type1 Diabetes are in part due to the longer duration of this disease, and early loss of insulin production. However if glucose is not well controlled, within 5 years, the Type II Diabetic often will develop complications. Why certain individuals develop this form of diabetes is unknown, but the genetic background is probably very different from Type 1 Diabetes. For instance, if one member of a pair of twins develops Type 2 diabetes, the other twin has a 95% chance of also developing this type of Diabetes. This fact rules out important contribution from the environment. <u>In contrast, a second twin develops Type 1 Diabetes only 25-50% of the time</u>, indicating that life situations (stress, infection, life style.) greatly contribute to the development of this form of the disease. Unfortunately, Diabetes is likely caused by the inheritance of *more than one* gene, which makes understanding the genetic background more difficult.

Certain features accelerate the development of Type II Diabetes. It is well established that *obesity predisposes individuals to the development of this disease.* Therefore, when a person has a strong family history of Type II Diabetes, he/she should maintain normal weight. This strategy will significantly delay or prevent the development of high blood glucose. A woman who is 5' 4" and medium build should weigh 120 lb or about 55 kilograms. To maintain her weight, she should consume 1600 calories each day. If she is 20 pounds (or about 10 kilograms) overweight, she should reduce her intake to 1100 calories each day. It is amazing how people deny the calories they consume each day. When I sit down with a patient and calculated the amount of calories consumed in a typical day's meals, you would think we were calculating the national debt. It is important for concerned people to weigh or measure their food and consult readily available tables to calculate calories in one's meals. They should keep a food diary. Lack of determining, or denial of the calories consumed is the single most common reason for failure of dieting here. The American Diabetes Association provides diets and how to measure calories, accessed on-line. New life-style changes include low amounts of calories ("alternate fasting") 2 days a week, 500 calories for women and 600 calories for men. The other days food calories should be as mentioned above. This combined with *regular exercise generating sweat* will certainly promote weight loss.

Certain stresses can accelerate the development of Diabetes. Severe injury, illness, or stress in one's life can enhance the diabetic process. Drugs, such as diuretics to control blood pressure or heart failure, or steroids like hydrocortisone pills can promote the development of Type II Diabetes. Sometimes, onset of Diabetes in later life can be the first indication of a new disease in that person. For instance, cancer of the pancreas is a very deadly, silent tumor, which often presents as Diabetes and weight loss. This occurs after the cancer replaces the normal, insulin-producing cells in the pancreas. Excessive production of hormones such as growth hormone or glucocorticoids like cortisol secreted by rare cancers can lead to elevated blood glucose.

Treatment of Type II Diabetes

Many of the strategies already mentioned for treatment of Type 1 Diabetes and prevention of the complications can be applied here. These include diet, exercise, and control of other diseases. Unique to Type 2 Diabetes is the widespread use of pill therapy in early stages, rather than insulin to control this disease.

Oral glucose-lowering medicines have been used for the treatment of Diabetes Mellitus for more than 50 years. The initial drugs approved were all sulfonylureas and currently this class includes drugs like glyburide, glipizide, and glimepiride. These drugs work mainly by increasing insulin secretion. A problem with these drugs is they are long lasting for hours and if an individual misses a meal then low blood glucose can occur. If hypoglycemia is not promptly treated, severe consequences could occur, including heart attack or coma. Glipizide causes a lower rate of hypoglycemia (low blood glucose). Also these drugs have side effects, including skin rashes, and occasionally interactions with other drugs, altering the effects of other medicines. If the individual takes a blood thinner, such as coumadin, both medicines should be adjusted by a physician. If a person has liver or kidney disease, adjustment in the dose of pill and insulin therapy may be needed. Sometimes a treatment must be abandoned especially if kidney function is low. Metformin is used in most patients if their kidney function is good and they don't have intestinal distress from taking the drug. This medication reduces development of large arterial disease and inhibits fasting hyperglycemia (elevated glucose).

After 10 years, approximately 50 % of Type II diabetics who are well controlled with pills will require insulin. This is primarily because the beta cells of the pancreas no longer make sufficient insulin. Individuals overwhelm the limited ability of the pancreas to secrete this hormone due to dietary excess. Recent work suggests the pancreatic insulin secreting cells don't die. Rather they change to a more primitive cell that does not make insulin. Interventional science is attempting to find a safe way to re-stimulate the cells to a mature pancreatic cell that secretes insulin.

New Generation of Drugs

Several new classes of drugs have been developed and are a step forward in controlling blood glucose. One class of drugs developed years ago includes pioglitazone or rosiglitazone. These drugs enhance the action of insulin, both produced by the pancreas or injected. As a result, an individual is less resistant to insulin. This lowers the HgbA1C and sometimes reduces the amount of injected insulin. This can also be used in Type 1 Diabetics. There can be some additional gain of weight from these pills but that can be controlled by a healthy lifestyle. Problems that do not allow using this class of medication is ongoing heart failure or significant edema (fluid often causes swelling of the legs).

More recently, a group of drugs that enhance insulin secretion from the pancreas, but only when eating. These drugs are now widely used. One group is DPP4 antagonists that increase insulin secretion only upon eating, acting as an incretin. Incretins are hormones in the intestine that stimulate release of more insulin from the pancreas *only* upon food entering the intestine. The problem of low glucose as mentioned for sulfonylurea drugs rarely happens with incretin-stimulating drugs.

Another class of drugs is related and are glucagon-like intestinal peptides (GLIP-1) that bind to a receptor in the intestines and has several beneficial effects not seen with the DPP4 antagonists. First this group of drugs inhibits glucagon secretion, the latter a hormone that acts on the liver to stimulate glucose release into the blood. The drug also stimulates incretin intestinal hormones to stimulate insulin secretion only upon eating a meal. This causes a decrease in the <u>post-meal glucose levels</u> that is often the key to good control of diabetes.

Additionally, this drug causes weight reduction of about 5-8%, the weight loss enhancing insulin action. This class of drugs has also been used to reduce weight in non-diabetics. This class of drugs has a long-term impact to lower serious heart and blood vessel disease occurrence or re-occurrence. This class of drugs (GLP1-agonist) has to be injected, once per week, but recently one member of this class, Semaglutide (Ozempic) can be given as pills or injection. More recently, a combination of a GLP1-agonist is being combined with GIP1, gastric inhibitory polypeptide, and this pill causes more weight loss and better glucose control. It has now been approved by the Food and Drug administration in the United States, for use especially in Type II Diabetes. This drug stimulates more insulin secretion and also is more potent to lose weight in overweight Diabetics, compared to GLIP-1 injection.

Another class of recent drugs is SGLT2 inhibitors. These pills cause the kidneys to excrete excess glucose into the urine. This is better than reabsorbing the urinary glucose, as it raises blood glucose levels. An example is Empaglifozin (Jardiance) given as a pill once per day. This drug has strong outcome effects to prevent progression of kidney disease and heart disease, such as heart failure and death from this cause. Blood pressure and weight (from excess fluid) can decrease from the use of these drugs. However, some individuals develop urinary tract infections (bladder and kidney). Also, this drug should not be given to Type 1 Diabetics because it can promote ketone-acidosis in this group, a dangerous situation. Also, patients with very severe kidney disease should not take this drug. Glucose levels in the blood significantly improve from taking this class of drugs.

Pregnancy and Diabetes Mellitus

When a woman becomes pregnant, a huge number of hormone changes occur. Many hormones are increasingly produced in the mother. This causes the proper environment for the development and growth of the fetus.

As pregnancy proceeds, increasingly greater secretion of growth promoting hormones results in resistance to the action of insulin. This is comparable to the basic problem in Type II Diabetes. However, the majority of woman can compensate for the relative insulin resistance, to maintain a normal blood glucose. Approximately 3-10 % of pregnant woman develop Gestational (pregnancy) diabetes. This disease is usually limited to the time of pregnancy. However as many as 50% of woman who develop high blood glucose during pregnancy, will become permanently diabetic over the following 5 years. This is especially found in obese women. At birth, the insulin resistance in the gestational diabetic mother almost immediately vanishes almost as the placenta is being expelled. How do we identify woman who eventually become diabetic during pregnancy? What are the current recommendations to strictly control blood glucose? Why is it important to do so? These issues are discussed in this section.

As a woman proceeds in her pregnancy, it is important to screen for abnormal glucose processing. Typically, a woman should have her urine measured for the presence of glucose and ketone bodies. Ketone formation is the body's response to insufficient glucose entering the cell. Since glucose is a critical fuel for cell function and development, the body will try to make its own glucose. This occurs to ensure normal fetal growth and development. A byproduct of manufacturing glucose in the body is the formation of ketones. If ketones and glucose are detected in the urine, this is a serious situation, requiring immediate evaluation by a physician knowledgeable about managing Gestational Diabetes.

Early identification and control of Gestational Diabetes is a major health area. The importance provides a strong justification for spending federal dollars on prenatal and maternal care. Unrecognized or poorly controlled Diabetes can be devastating, particularly for the fetus. As a result of insulin resistance, more insulin is secreted, which acts as a growth factor for the unborn child. At delivery, these children can be physically huge, and have poorly developed, enlarged hearts, kidneys, lungs, and other organs. They have poor muscle tone at birth and delayed or permanently impaired muscle development. The babies can have large tongues, which in difficult births can block the baby's airway and produce brain damage due to lack of oxygen. The offspring can be born prematurely and suffer from immaturity of the lungs, leading to respiratory distress. They often have lower IQ scores then children from non-diabetic mothers.

If a woman is found to have glucose in her urine, her blood glucose is measured, and if elevated, therapy is begun. If the blood glucose is not elevated, a glucose tolerance test is performed during weeks 24-28. Here, blood glucose is measured 1 and 2 hours after a woman drinks a liquid sweetened with 50-75 grams of glucose. Fasting glucose should be 95-105 mg/dl, and post meal or post glucose tolerance test, the 1 and 2 hour measurements should not exceed 140. If a woman is diagnosed from this test as having gestational Diabetes (more than 140), treatment is started. First, the woman is placed on a diet which is sufficient to provide nutrition to the baby, It is also important to control blood glucose. This is usually 1800-2500 calories a day unless the mother is obese and calories are diminished to 1300 calories, less than 30% as fat. Exercise is also instituted. If this does not strictly control the blood glucose, then insulin is added for the remainder of the pregnancy as the standard care. Fasting blood glucose is usually controlled between 60-100 mg.

After a woman gives birth, there is usually no insulin resistance and injected insulin usually can be stopped. The woman is then followed for signs of developing Diabetes later in life. A large study of gestational diabetics indicates that taking rosiglitazone or pioglitazone can prevent development of diabetes later in life by as much as 80 percent, Overall, the control of the mother's metabolic state can have significant positive effects for the fetus. Good control prevents enlargement of the newborn baby, altered metabolism, and prevents obesity that can persist into child and adulthood.

Conclusions

Our understanding of the causes of Diabetes has greatly improved, though still incomplete. Only by understanding the nature of this disease can recommendations be made to prevent or delay the development of Diabetes. New methods of treatment will allow for earlier and more natural control of blood glucose. Preventing many of the complications which plague the diabetic also reduces the development of premature death. In the future, the artificial pancreas will be used to better control blood glucose. For better control now, insulin pumps regulated by controlling glucose monitors represents a step forward for reducing hyperglycemia. Cure of the disease awaits the selective and normal expression of the insulin gene or pancreatic stem cells implanted in the pancreas.

Thyroid and Parathyroid
Health and Disease

Introduction

Thyroid hormones are made and secreted by the thyroid gland in the neck. The process of incorporating iodine into thyroglobulin protein creates a final hormone product of the gland, thyroxine. Interestingly, people who live in areas in many countries that have very low amounts of iodine salt in their diet (not America) can result in an enlarged thyroid gland (goiter) and hypothyroid state. Mainly thyroxine (T4) is secreted from healthy glands with a smaller amount of triiodothyronine (T3) made and secreted from the gland. However, more often T3 is made from action of proteins that convert T4 to T3 in numerous organs in the body. In the hypothalamus part of the brain, a hormone called TRH is secreted that stimulates TSH production in the pituitary gland, at the base of the skull, TSH is secreted into the blood and then binds to its protein receptors in the thyroid gland, ultimately stimulating thyroid hormone secretion.

Importantly, T3 is the stronger hormone (3-4 times the strength of T4) but much more T4 is secreted from healthy thyroid glands, making up the difference during normal health. T3 acts rapidly and binds its receptor more strongly, thus being a stronger hormone when compared to the same amount of T4. This becomes more important in disease states that are described below. The effects of thyroid hormones are seen in many organs in the body, and especially in the central nervous system (brain and nerve systems), the heart and arteries system, and bones. The positive effects at normal levels of thyroid hormone are overcome by excessive or decreased amounts from disease states of the thyroid, with strong results for the systems mentioned.

In pregnancy, thyroid hormones in the mother are increased in production. This is most important in the first 3 months of pregnancy when the fetus can't make its own thyroid hormones, thus depending on the mother's T4 and T3. After that, the fetus manufactures its own thyroid hormones. In general, it is mothers with a family history of thyroid disease that are most likely to develop thyroid disorders during pregnancy. Thyroid hormone is very important for normal brain development, both in the fetus while in the uterus and in the newborn baby during the first years of life. Thus, it is important for both mother and the newborn child to be euthyroid (normal), the newborn being tested for low thyroid function at birth. If the mother develops hyperthyroidism, a drug called Propylthiouracil can be given in the first trimester of pregnancy, then Methimazole is substituted in the remainder of pregnancy, as needed. If the drugs cause problems in the mother, surgical removal of the mother's thyroid can be done in the second trimester but only in an emergent situation. If hypothyroid, the mother is given Synthroid (T4) to produce normal pregnant levels in the mother for the remainder of pregnancy. Some of the T4 is transferred to the fetus.

Common Thyroid Diseases

Hypothyroidism

A common disease in men and women is hypothyroidism. This is where the thyroid gland does not produce normal levels of T4. Most often this happens due to malfunction of the gland, often due to antibodies that attack the thyroid. This causes inflammation and resulting destruction of the thyroid gland. Hashimotos thyroiditis (inflammation) is the most common cause of hypothyroidism. As mentioned, a lack of iodine in the diet can also lead to low levels of T4. This does not happen commonly in the United States because most food has iodine salt.

Blood testing reveals low T4 and elevated TSH in most hypothyroidism. The TSH is high because the pituitary gland where TSH is made senses the low T4. So the pituitary adjusts and secretes more TSH to stimulate the thyroid gland. However as mentioned the thyroid is not functioning properly. So, doctors will give Synthroid to these people, resulting in normal levels of T4 and TSH. Associated symptoms should resolve. Typical symptoms are fatigue and weakness, dry skin, constipation, and sensitivity to cold. Thinking can be abnormal, moderate weight gain, and muscle cramps can occur. Hair can be brittle and menstrual periods are often heavy.

When replacing the loss of T4 production, we aim to keep the blood levels in the mid-normal range. This is especially important in older individuals who may have osteoporosis that can be enhanced by too much T4 replacement. Also, individuals with a history or strong likelihood to develop cardiac arrythmias should be at the lower range of normal from replacement treatment. That is because too much thyroid hormone can stimulate severe arrythmias. Some patients have hypothalamus or pituitary disease resulting in a low TSH, causing low T4 production. Further investigation is needed to rule out other decreased pituitary hormone and resulting disease. This includes ACTH from the pituitary that stimulates cortisol secretion from the two adrenal glands that lie on top of the kidneys. Low ACTH results in low cortisol production.

One common consult to Endocrinologists is for possible subclinical hypothyroidism. This is a situation where the T4 levels are low normal and the TSH is moderately elevated but the patients have no complaints that are consistent with full hypothyroidism. If the patient progresses where the TSH is now above 10 to stimulate and maintain normal T4 levels, we provide the thyroxine (T4) medication at that point. Other causes of subclinical or clinical hypothyroidism include a drug, amiodarone, that is used to inhibit heart arrythmias. This drug can also cause hyperthyroidism in some individuals. Cancer patients receiving immune check point drugs can also develop either hypothyroidism or hyperthyroidism.

Hyperthyroidism

The most common form is *Grave's disease*, where antibodies to the thyroid gland cells stimulate thyroid hormone synthesis. This causes excessive T3 and T4 secreted into the blood and therefore into to many body organs. compared to the normal state. There are many possible symptoms, including moist and smooth skin, heat intolerance, weight loss, strong reflexes, and increased heart rate (sometimes arrythmias like atrial fibrillation). The latter can be problematic. Anxiety and irritability can occur. Sleep can be disturbed causing fatigue. Muscles can be weak and multiple daily-bowel movements can occur. Blood level measurements of T4 and T3 levels are elevated and TSH is usually very low. A closely related hyperthyroid state is *Hashitoxicosis*, presenting similarly. Finally some drugs mentioned in causing hypothyroidism can also stimulate the thyroid gland. Treatment of hyperthyroidism can be done through multiple ways.

Commonly used drugs that block hyperthyroidism in pregnancy (Propylthiouracil and Methimazole) are often used in Grave's disease and the other causes of hyperthyroidism. The drugs can be used often for many years if necessary; sometimes the gland restores normal function after several months and the medications are stopped. Another treatment is administering radioactive iodine that is strongly taken up by the thyroid gland and results in the death of thyroid gland cells. This reduces excess thyroid hormone synthesis to a normal level. However, over time the gland undergoes significant damage and often become hypothyroid. T4 pills are given to restore normal amounts of thyroid hormone, as with hypothyroidism. The least used intervention is surgical removal of the thyroid gland. An experienced surgeon is important for performing the operation

There is also a state of subclinical hyperthyroidism. Here there are no or few symptoms of hyperthyroidism. However the blood TSH is very low and T4 is high normal or slightly elevated. Subclinical hyperthyroidism is most often treated with the anti-thyroid drugs mentioned above until normal lab results return. Another cause of hyperthyroidism is thyroiditis. This is when the gland releases a lot of thyroid hormone usually for a relatively short time. The common forms are in the mother after giving birth, *post-partum thyroiditis*, and this is treated temporarily with the drugs mentioned. If the heart rate is rapid, a beta-blocker like metoprolol is added to restore a normal rate. Also this can occur when a virus causes inflammation of the thyroid. Usually this lasts for about a week as *subacute thyroiditis*. If the inflammation is severe, hydrocortisone can be given with or without beta-blockers. Most of the time, anti-thyroid drugs are not necessary here. Virus-caused thyroiditis diminishes to normal gland function and rarely recurs.

Thyroid Cancer

Thyroid cancer is most often relatively benign, meaning it does not usually metastasize to other organs. It rarely causes hypo or hyperthyroidism. The presentation is often a nodule in the thyroid that is discovered by imaging of the neck and chest done for other reasons, The nodule can undergo a thin needle biopsy at an Endocrinologist's office; this determines whether the nodule is harmless or a malignancy. If cancer, a very experienced surgeon should remove the nodule and often at least the thyroid lobe (left or right half of the gland based on where the nodule is). Sometimes the entire thyroid is removed if the nodule is cancerous and several of the sampled lymph nodes in the neck also show cancer. After full thyroid removal, radioactive Iodine is given to be taken up in the neck to destroy any tumor that is still present. Both remaining normal and cancer cells usually express the protein that takes up the iodine into the cells. Using radioactive iodine as treatment kills the remaining cancer and normal cells. However, advanced cancer often loses the ability to take up iodine thus not responding to this cancer treatment. Thus this treatment after surgery is not used.

I131 killing remaining cancer and normal cells is important to prevent cancer recurrence. The individual is also given thyroid hormone replacement with T4 if the entire thyroid gland is removed. T4 inhibits growth of remaining cancer cells not removed by surgery or I131 treatment. T4 provides normal thyroid levels for body functions in the patient. Also, any normal cells that remain can confuse the situation. Blood levels of the protein thyroglobulin are used to determine the state of possible tumor recurrence or normal cells remaining in the neck. Measuring thyroglobulin is important. This produces determination of whether there is a need for additional therapy. Also, this measurement suggests the tumor is present or has invaded the lung or other organs. That requires PET scanning images to determine if there is thyroid cancer spreading to other organs, requiring further treatment.

One form of thyroid cancer is called Medullary Carcinoma. This is often inherited in families by a genetic predisposition due to mutations of the RET gene. This thyroid cancer can be identified in very early stages of development in children from families that have this genetic syndrome. Identification results in surgical removal of the thyroid gland for cure. This is part of a multi-organ syndrome called MEN2, and includes pheochromocytoma that can be a tumor in several organs in the body, even if usually not a typical cancer can cause very high blood pressure. In addition, benign parathyroid tumors usually are often found. Parathyroid cancer is very rare, and the benign adenoma does not spread to other parts of the body The adenomas secrete parathyroid hormone in excess, creating hyperparathyroidism (see below),

Parathyroid hormone function and disease

Surrounding the thyroid gland in the neck lies four small glands that secrete parathyroid hormone (PTH). This hormone regulates calcium levels in the blood and tissues. This occurs in part by PTH stimulating production of the most potent form of vitamin D,1,25-di-hydroxy vitamin D. This 1.25 form of vitamin D increases calcium in blood and organs. This occurs partly by increasing re-absorbing of calcium from urine in the kidney and absorption of calcium in the intestine from food such as dairy products. This form of vitamin D and the resulting higher calcium together normally inhibit PTH secretion keeping normal levels of calcium.

The ability to make this form of vitamin D is severely decreased in advanced kidney diseases, resulting in low calcium. Also, in kidney failure, it is often important to decrease excessive amounts of PTH that occurs. Reducing PTH decreases its resorbing action on bone. As a result, there is a decrease of advanced osteoporosis and fracture risk. Normal levels of 1.25-hydroxy Vitamin D stimulate bone forming cells, named the osteoblast.

Excess production of PTH occurs when one of the four glands undergoes transition to a benign adenoma that oversecretes PTH. In most people as calcium becomes high, PTH secretion is decreased. However, the PTH-secreting adenomas are not well suppressed by the resulting high calcium levels. The approach in younger and middle-aged individuals is to surgically remove the usual one adenoma as a cure for hyperparathyroidism, important especially in individuals that have osteoporosis or calcium kidney stones.

Occasionally, all four glands undergo enlargement that also produces hyperparathyroidism. In individuals with advanced kidney disease, the PTH levels can be very high and a drug called Cinacalcet can reduce the elevated calcium and PTH levels. In parathyroid adenoma-caused hyperparathyroidism that can occur from kidney disease, Cinacalcet is used. Especially this drug is used if the individual can't undergo adenoma surgical removal. Finally, *very rarely parathyroid cancer occurs*, presenting with extremely high calcium and PTH levels. If posible to surgically remove the cancer, that is the best option for treatment.

Bone Diseases

Formation and growth of bone is a fundamental part of development. The so-called growing pains in teenagers can be real and result from a rapid increase in the length and size of bones, stimulated by sex hormones (estrogen and testosterone) during early puberty. *Why are some individuals, like Kareem Abdul-Jabbar or Shaquille O'Neal more than 7 foot tall while jockeys like Eddie Shoemaker are barely 5 foot?* The answer is each person's bone cells respond differently to the growth factors and sex hormones which cause lengthening of bone. This probably is due to unique gene makeup of each person that we don't currently understand.

As one ages, the process of bone formation changes, and diseases of bone result from abnormal bone growth and remodeling. In this chapter, the important metabolic bone diseases, include Osteoporosis, Rickets that are also named Osteomalacia, and Paget's disease and these will be discussed. A basic understanding of bone formation and how to enhance this process and preserve bone mass is provided.

Bone Growth

As children, we were repetitively reminded (or is it plagued) by our parents to drink lots of milk, because otherwise we wouldn't grow tall. In fact, the calcium, vitamin D and other minerals contained in milk are important for normal bone development. Does this mean that Herve Villachez, star of the TV series *Fantasy Island*, is a dwarf because he didn't drink milk as a child, and so his bones didn't fully grow? Or, is there a genetic program, unique to each of us, that dictates how our bone cells use the raw materials for bone formation? What determines the ultimate length and development of bones? Are diseases of bone formation which occur as we age unalterable? To answer these questions, it is important to know something about the composition and process of bone formation. Bone is made up of minerals and protein (collagen). This combination gives bone the strength of metal yet provides flexibility and support at the joints of the body, like our knees and elbows.

The mineral content of bone is made up mainly of calcium and phosphorous, which are used to form bone by a cell called the osteoblast. Mineral is deposited and fills in the protein skeleton in mature bone. This is similar to a child coloring in pictures which are already outlined in a coloring book.

As the bone is mineralized, the mature osteoblast cell stops functioning, and is enclosed in the mature bone, and further formation is taken up by newly formed osteoblasts. The role of this cell is not very different from the worker bee in the beehive, whose sole purpose is to construct the honeycomb. At the completion of his job, the worker bee like the osteoblast dies and is encased in the comb itself becoming immortalized as part of its accomplishment.

Bone growth in children is carried out slightly differently, but in all situations, a second cell, the Osteoclast, serves as the Michelangelo of bone formation. The Osteoclast resorbs bone, molding and shaping newly formed bone, removing dead bone, and generally serving a housekeeping function (there is no equivalent to washing windows). *It is important to make the distinctions between bone forming and bone remodeling cells,* because understanding the diseases of bone formation or tactics to treat bone disease depends on this distinction.

The bone forming and bone resorbing/remodeling processes are normally tightly related. Un-coupling of this relationship can result in bone diseases, such as Osteoporosis or Osteomalacia, the two most common bone diseases affecting the population of the United States today. Ella Fitzgerald, the beloved jazz singer, was hospitalized shortly before her death. She suffered a fracture of the head of the long bone of the leg, the femur, where it fits into the hip socket. Former president Gerald Ford had both knees replaced, and football injuries likely contributed to his problem. These famous people and millions of other Americans are victims of the most common form of bone disease, Osteoporosis. Non-coordinated activity of the Osteoblast and Osteoclast results in unstable bone in these people. The unstable bone is vulnerable to fracture after trivial accidents or even without any trauma.

Hormonal Control of Bone Formation

What regulates the activity of these two bone cells? Hormones become very important. One hormone, called Calcitonin, is a protein made in specialized cells of the thyroid gland. This hormone inhibits the bone resorbing actions of the Osteoclast. In this way, the body can control excessive bone destruction or regulate bone sculpting. This knowledge has led to the use of synthetic Calcitonin to treat diseases which are the result of too much bone resorption. For instance, the high calcium level resulting from bone destruction in some cancers has been typically treated with Calcitonin. More recently, more potent drugs are used instead to treat bones that are targeted in some cancers, discussed below.

Excess bone resorption plays an important role in Osteoporosis. Newer drugs have been developed in the last few years that strongly inhibit the action of the Osteoclast. The bisphosphonates are a class of drugs used for treating cancer-related elevations of calcium, and severe Osteoporosis and Paget's diseases of bone. Their role will be discussed more thoroughly.

Other hormones also play a regulatory role. Parathyroid hormone (PTH) is made in four small glands in the neck and plays a major role in absorbing calcium and phosphorous from the diet, through the intestine. As mentioned, PTH stimulates production of the active form of Vitamin D by the kidney, from a less active form made in the liver. Active vitamin D is necessary for calcium and phosphorous absorption from the intestine and kidney. In this way, the parathyroid, liver, and kidney all contribute to calcium-phosphorous balance in the body. This is crucial to bone formation. Parathyroid hormone also indirectly stimulates the osteoclast to resorb bone, and therefore people who secrete excess PTH (hyperparathyroidism) may have bone disease and calcium kidney stones. Parathyroid levels can be excessive from secretion from a benign tumor (adenoma) of one or more of the parathyroid glands. This can be surgically removed for cure and prevention of accelerated Osteoporosis in some individuals.

Low vitamin D levels also lead to increased parathyroid hormone (PTH) secretion as a compensation. This can be corrected by taking Vitamin D pills to normalize blood levels of this vitamin, at a level of 30-40.ng/ml. Calcium intake is important to bone health and is attained through consuming dairy products and leafy vegetables. Supplementation by calcium pills should be used only if blood calcium levels are low. Low calcium is most often due to avoidance of dairy products. However, upon aging, many individuals are unable to digest dairy products (milk, cheese, yogurt) because of the loss of the enzyme in our intestine that degrades the milk sugar, lactose. The loss of this enzyme, known as lactase deficiency, promotes bloating, belching, abdominal pain, breaking wind and diarrhea after eating ice cream or drinking milk. Such individuals quickly learn to avoid dairy products if they have any desire to be in a public place.

The result of lactose intolerance is the intake of calcium and vitamin D is severely restricted, which leads to a lack of mineral to build new bones. The lack of calcium in the diet of middle aged and elderly Americans is made worse by the inability to properly absorb calcium through the intestine, because of a lower production of the active form of vitamin D. Combined with the accelerated rate of bone breakdown, this leads to a negative calcium balance and decreased bone density. To make up for the lack of dairy products in the diet, many people swallow a daily dose of vitamins and calcium. The current recommendations for all people is to have 1500 mg of calcium in the daily diet, or obtained through calcium pills, with vitamin D, 50,000 units, once per week for a month to correct a deficit. Then, Vitamin D at 1500-2000 units per day is sufficient to maintain normal levels. Vitamin D3 is the best form of this vitamin to take.

Many other protein and steroid hormones affect bone cells and bone development, but their mechanisms and contributions to disease are often not as clear. Thyroid hormone, when produced in excess or given in too large replacement doses in hypothyroid individuals, can cause additional bone resorption and promote possible fractures.

Elderly women often have very low bone mass. The bone mass from minerals in the bone is determined by a simple scanning test of several bones in our body. It is called a DEXA scan of the bone. These same women may have low thyroid activity (hypothyroid) and require replacement thyroid hormone. These women should receive the lowest effective treatment dose possible to avoid enhanced bone resorption and thereby prevent fractures.

Individuals receiving glucocorticoids (cortisone, dexamtheasome) for lung disease such as asthma; or for various forms of arthritis or other diseases, should be given the lowest doses of these steroids. This is because cortisone and other glucocorticoids cause bone resorption. In addition, locally produced bone growth factors play a major role in bone disease. We do not know how to manipulate these bone and cartilage growth factors to work strongly.

At our annual family picnic, I noticed that Aunt Sara was progressively shrinking. As a child, I was told that this was because I was growing taller, and so it only seemed that my aunt was shorter. In fact, she had lost several inches of height due to collapse of several bones in her spinal column from Osteoporosis.

Osteoporosis

Osteoporosis is a bone disorder showing impaired bone formation and increased resorption. This leads to a decrease in the amount of total bone because bone resorption is greater than bone formation especially in older women. In Osteoporosis, the bone *mineral quality* is normal but emerging evidence indicates bone strength and structure are abnormal. Most hip fractures in the elderly population are the result of Osteoporosis. The person suffering from this disease has no obvious symptoms until a fracture occurs. Pain, arthritis, or limitation of motion are not part of *this* disease until late in the course. A person may find out that he or she has this disease because they had an x-ray for unrelated reasons, and the radiologist noted that the bones were "washed out" (demineralized). Then a DEXA scan of the bones determines whether treatment should be started.

Why is Osteoporosis a public health concern? According to the National Osteoporosis Foundation (NOF), in the United States in 2015, individuals over age 65 developed 2.3 million fractures due to Osteoporosis. Within a year of an Osteoporotic fracture, 15% of these individuals suffer at least one additional fracture and nearly 20% died. Mortality was highest with hip fracture, where 30% die in the following year. In 2018 it was estimated that 10.2 million adults in the United States have Osteoporosis, and an additional 43.4 million have low bone mass as a prelude to Osteoporosis. Osteoporosis results in 1/3rd of all women over 65 having spinal column bone fractures. One woman in three over the age of 75 has a hip fracture, and the figures are not much better for older males. The costs of Osteoporosis-related fracture are estimated at 3 billion dollars yearly.

The natural history of bone growth and loss is important. Peak bone mass (the total amount of bone in the body) is reached by age 30 and begins to decrease soon after. The annual loss of bone mass at that time is less than one-half percent per year, and is maintained steadily as males age. In women, there is accelerated loss after menopause. During the 10 years following the end of menstruation, a woman can lose up to 20% of her bone mass (including the long bones and the spinal column vertebral bone). Fracturing occurs after 25% of peak bone mass has been lost.

The process itself changes after menopause because the osteoclast becomes extremely active. A major contributor is loss of estrogen produced in the ovaries after menopause. *Loss of estrogen* after menopause causes increased bone resorption (by the osteoclast). Also, loss of estrogen results in fewer bone forming cells, osteoblasts, causing decreased bone formation in addition to the accelerated bone loss. Estrogen also acts as a border patrolman, preventing parathyroid hormone from gaining access to the bone. Men do not have a comparable loss of sex hormone (testosterone) production in middle age. The similar protective effect of the male sex hormone, testosterone, prevents accelerated bone loss. Interestingly, 75% of the bone protection by testosterone in men is due to conversion of testosterone to estrogen in the body. Estrogen prevents the increased level of bone disease, both in men and in women, until men are older than 70 years of age. This is because testosterone levels decrease in *advanced* age in men, also reducing estrogen formation from the testosterone. Thus I always tell men to get in touch with their feminine side as it is mainly estrogen that preserves their bone.

Men often have a larger bone mass to begin with and they lack the accelerated loss that occurs upon menopause in women. So, a decline in bone mass is not as devastating. Interestingly, both black men and women have a larger bone mass than Caucasians, and therefore have less severe bone disease with aging. Also, obese individuals often have less bone loss. This is probably because fat cells can produce estrogen which slows down the bone loss process.

As mentioned, some medications such as glucocorticoids and excessive thyroid hormone, or long-term use of the blood thinner, heparin, can result in Osteoporosis and fractures. In some elderly people, the kidney is diseased and can't produce the active form of vitamin D that is necessary for calcium and phosphorous absorption from food. To compensate, a greater secretion of parathyroid hormone occurs. This results in accelerated removal of calcium from the bone and altered bone production. This cycle of events leads to increased bone destruction.

Life-style can also affect the rate of bone loss. Clearly, regular weight bearing exercise decreases the rate of loss of bone density. Exercise applies stress to bone which stimulates the process of bone formation and prevents resorption. Cigarette smoking accelerates bone loss, and heavy alcohol intake can lead to Osteoporosis. In part this happens because the alcoholic doesn't eat enough foods high in minerals and vitamins when drinking.

Not all forms of Osteoporosis are the result of the aging process. Rather, Osteoporosis may be the first sign of a previously unsuspected, underlying disease. A disease of bone marrow cells which leads to a cancer called Multiple Myeloma can present in early stages as Osteoporosis. Interestingly, the Myeloma cell makes a protein which acts directly on the bone to cause bone resorption by the osteoclast, leading to thinning and fractures. This results in the blood levels of calcium becoming very elevated and high calcium in the blood leads to constipation, weakness, and excessive urination as symptoms.

Other diseases frequently associated with Osteoporosis include excess production of cortisone by the adrenal gland. (Cushings disease). Also any disease that causes loss of male or female sex hormone production has the same effects. Unchecked, diseases of the stomach and intestine that limit absorption of vitamin D, calcium, and phosphorous can contribute. Liver disease, lung disease and rare inherited bone diseases can each lead to Osteoporosis. Identifying and treating the underlying cause is important in preventing progression.

Recommendations

Prevention

What can be done to prevent the loss of bone with aging? Exercising regularly especially weight bearing exercise, like walking/running. Also, stopping smoking, and drinking alcohol in moderation is a strategy for preventing many diseases, including Osteoporosis. Daily intake of calcium and vitamin D in the diet is important. As mentioned earlier, eating leafy vegetables and consuming milk can provide this intake. Milk can be purchased with the protein lactobacillus acidophilus which digests the milk sugar, lactose. This prevents lactose intolerance in some people, and does not produce intestinal symptoms as does regular milk in some people. Yogurt, which contains less undigested lactose, can be a solution. Unfortunately, some commercial manufacturers sweeten yogurt with *lactose* and therefore, the label must be examined for presence of this sugar. Calcium supplementation with calcium carbonate tablets daily provides sufficient calcium if *dietary intake* of calcium and vitamin D doesn't occur. Women might take estrogen and progesterone supplementation after menopause to help prevent accelerated bone loss.

How does one know that they are developing accelerated bone loss? This information can be obtained from the DEXA scanning. This sophisticated technique quantifies bone mass, comparing your mass to the general population. This scan gives your physician important information to begin a program to prevent the ravages of extreme bone mineral loss and fractures. Adopting a healthy lifestyle as mentioned greatly aids in preventing development of significant Osteoporosis.

Treatment of Osteoporosis

Stopping bone loss from resorption

What are the currently available treatments for the person who has developed significant Osteoporosis, without or with resulting fractures? If bone loss is the result of an underlying disease, treating that disease may reverse the resorption process. This would prevent fractures. Taking vitamin D and calcium if you are deficient limits the extent of Osteoporosis. Using estrogen as detailed, further development of Osteoporosis is strongly limited. This helps to prevent bone fractures.

Most specific medical treatments focus on decreasing bone resorption. Drugs or synthetic hormones that limit osteoclast-caused resorption of bone are the main form of treatment. The bisphosphonate group of drugs may be useful as pills or by injection. Oral bisphosphonates such as Alendronate (Fosamax) can be given once per week.

More recent drugs work through different mechanisms to inhibit osteoclast resorption of bone. Zolendronic Acid (Reclast) is given by intravenous infusion over 20 minutes, and as an out-patient at an infusion clinic This is given once every 12 months and no other anti-resorption medication is required in between infusions. That is because Zolendronic acid is stored in the bone. There are minimal side effects of infusion that can be prevented by taking Tylenol at the time of infusion.

A second drug is injected under the skin. This is Prolia (denosumab), an antibody that blocks activity of the osteoclast, thereby preserving the bone. This drug is injected once every six months and is especially useful in individuals that have moderate kidney disease. The drug is also used in women who are being treated for breast cancer by taking *estrogen inhibitory treatment*. Prolia is also used in men who take drugs that inhibit testosterone to prevent progression of prostate cancer. This drug is used to prevent or treat Osteoporosis. With the cancers mentioned, Prolia can limit metastases of these cancers to bone. Zolendronic Acid infusion is also used in individuals who have cancer such as Multiple Myeloma that often causes high calcium levels in the blood,. This drug often reduces the high calcium levels, while the underlying cancer is being treated.

For relatively mild osteoporosis, the pills are a good way to proceed. Prolia or Zolendronic acid are used in more serious Osteoporosis especially if fractures have occurred in the hip or vertebral bones that make up the spine. Also the ability of the various drugs to prevent bone fractures is very different.

Table 1-Ability of available anti-resorption treatments to *prevent fractures* in high at-risk individuals

Drug	Vertebral fracture	Hip	Wrist
Fosamax	50% reduced	36%	36%
Prolia	75% reduced	50%	50%
Zolendronic Acid	75% reduced	50%	50%

In the post-menopausal woman taking replacement estrogen and progesterone (the latter to prevent uterine cancer that can be caused by estrogen alone), estrogen prevents Osteoporosis and fractures, approximately equivalent to Fosamax. Similarly, raloxifene or the combination of estrogen and bazedoxifene (manufactured by Pfizer) also prevents bone fractures, equivalent to estrogen treatment. There is no enhanced prevention by combining estrogen with one of the other anti-resorption medications mentioned.

When an individual has taken pills for 5 years and injection for 3 years, and the osteoporosis then is not severe, there may be a "drug holiday" where individuals can stop the treatment for 3-5 years. The bone density is checked by DEXA scan after 12 months of holiday to make sure there is no significant bone loss.

Upon long time use of the drugs by an individual, atypical hip fractures or disease of the jaw bone can occur. However, these are not common and the positive effects of protection against standard fractures of many bones greatly outweighs the very small risk of developing atypical fractures especially. The recommendations from the Osteoporosis and Endocrine Societies are to use the anti-resorptive drugs mentioned, preventing typical fractures.

Bone formation

Another approach is to build additional bone especially in someone who has very severe Osteoporosis and has fractured or is at high risk of fracture in the future. The first such medication is a short form of parathyroid hormone (PTH), the first 34 amino acids of the hormone, called Teriparatide. This is injected under the skin once every day for two years to get maximal benefit. This includes causing strengthening of all bones and increasing the mineral content of the bone. The Dexa scan usually shows strong improvement at 2 years. One would hope that using Teriparatide plus an anti-resorption drug like Alendronate would be the best treatment but unfortunately the combination was no better than each medicine given one, then the other, and not at the same time. So the bone forming agent is given first for 2 years, and is then followed by up to 5 years of using just an antiresorptive drug, A drug holiday is then often started if the Dexa scan is good and no fractures have occurred.

A newer anabolic that is a bone forming drug is Abaloparatide that is given by injection daily under the skin for 2 years, followed by an antiresorptive medication as described. Currently, an Abaloparatide skin patch is being developed but not yet available. This synthetic protein is a close cousin to parathyroid hormone. There is one trial that showed using Alendronate and Abaloparatide <u>together</u> is better than each one by itself sequentially, in terms of fracture reduction. Both Teriparatide and Abaloparatide caused an 85% reduction in vertebral fractures, and a 43% reduction in all other fractures (hip, wrist, etc.). Again these drugs should be used in those at very high risk for fracture (very concerning Dexa scan score) and/or a history of multiple fractures despite other treatment.

The most recent drug approved and in use is Romosozumab. This is used in women with severe osteoporosis (low T-score more negative than -2.5 and a history of fractures). This drug is taken once per month by injection under the skin for 1 year. Currently this drug is not recommended for women who have a history of heart damage or stroke. This drug both builds bone and prevents bone resorption. Its main function is to block the effect of the protein sclerostin that prevents new bone formation. In clinical trials this drug seems to build more bone than the previously mentioned bone-forming drugs. After one year, Romososumab should be replaced by Alendronate or another anti-resorptive drug. As an overall result, there is a 75% reduction in vertebral fractures and a 38% reduction in hip fractures after the follow up 1 year of Alendronate.

New drugs and approaches from research to prevent fractures are ongoing. If not successful, the public truly will have (dare I say it), *a bone to pick* with the research and pharmaceutical communities.

Osteomalacia

Osteomalacia is another bone disease due to decreased mineral content of bone. If you looked at such bone under a microscope, the lack of calcium and phosphorous would be striking.

Tests of bone chemistry show these individuals almost always have very low phosphorous and low normal or low calcium levels in their blood. A bone protein, alkaline phosphatase, is almost always elevated and serves as a marker for Osteomalacia.

Osteomalacia is perhaps best known for the misery it caused in Charles Dickens' 19th century England. There were few child labor laws at that time, and in urban areas, youngsters and their parents worked long hours, rarely seeing the sun, and omitting dairy products from their diet. Sunlight is critical for the first step in producing the active form of vitamin D. It has been estimated that 5 minutes of noon sunlight daily is all that is required for *activation* of Vitamin D that we get from what we eat and drink. These children received neither proper nutrition, nor exposure to the sun and developed the disease known as Rickets, a form of Osteomalacia.

Rickets produces short, malformed individuals whose bones are deformed and weak, and easy fracturing is common. Several medical conditions can lead to Osteomalacia. A frequent cause is poor intestine absorption of vitamins and phosphorous and calcium.

Malabsorption is the inability of the intestine to normally absorb fat and vitamins and can be caused by chronic diarrhea, parasites, lymphoma of the intestine, or loss of pancreas function. The pancreas makes proteins that are important for intestinal absorption of food and nutrients. The inability to absorb vitamin D can lead to Osteomalacia. After Vitamin D is absorbed and is actively modified by the sun, it is transported to the liver and kidney for complete activation. This is also required for calcium absorption in our intestines and contributes to bone formation. Therefore, diseases which impair the functions of the liver and kidney can lead to

Osteomalacia. Some people who take phenobarbital and dilantin pills to prevent epilepsy can also suffer from this bone disease. It can be treated with vitamin D pills.

Another group of diseases which cause Osteomalacia are due to the loss of phosphorous through the urine, or as mentioned, the inability to absorb phosphorous from the intestine. An inherited disease which impairs phosphorous intestinal absorption and increases phosphorous wasting is called phosphate diabetes (not involving glucose) or X chromosome-linked low phosphorous rickets (Don't worry, this will never appear in the New York Times crossword puzzle). Males are afflicted with this disease and often have bow-legs, bone pain, and fractures at an early age. Treatment with active vitamin D and phosphorous can be used to lessen the severity of disease. Various diseases of the kidney can also lead to phosphate loss in the urine. In certain families, rickets can be caused by an abnormality of the ability of vitamin D to bind to its protein receptor in various tissues, including the intestine and bone. It has been found that the receptor protein is mutated (abnormal) in these individuals, or that the chemical events following vitamin D binding are impaired.

This represents an example where an abnormal interaction of a hormone with its receptor is responsible for a disease. This is a mechanism for instance where a physical appearing woman is genetically a man. But if testosterone can't bind a mutated receptor inherited from birth, this person develops as a woman because of the lack of testosterone action. Also, testosterone is converted to estrogen in all normal men also. Here testosterone is not working properly but the estrogen is working properly so the man physically looks like a woman.

In the elderly, Osteoporosis and Osteomalacia can co-exist in approximately 20% of affected people. Bone or muscle aching is a sign that Osteomalacia exists, and both disorders need investigation and treatment. Importantly, diseases of the kidney, liver, intestine or parathyroid gland can promote either Osteoporosis or Osteomalacia. It is not well understood why one form of bone disease occurs over another. The decrease in serum phosphorous plus bone pain should alert doctors to Osteomalacia that is not as common as Osteoporosis. Arthritis pain should not be mistaken for the bone pain of Osteomalacia.

Treatment

The treatment of established Osteomalacia involves correcting the underlying disease if possible. Providing adequate vitamin D, in its active form (1,25 hydroxy Vitamin D), calcium, and sometimes phosphorous pills often greatly improves and sometimes cures the Osteomalacia.

Paget's Disease

This disease commonly occurs in the elderly white population. Its incidence is estimated to be as high as 3% of all Caucasians over the age of 55. But most of the time there are no symptoms so there is no investigation or diagnosis. One of the major theories as to why Beethoven became deaf is that the composer developed advanced Paget's disease. The cause of Paget's disease is unknown, although chronic virus infection of the Osteoclast bone-resorbing cell is a leading theory.

Curiously, this disease is characterized by *both* excessive bone formation <u>and</u> bone resorption. It's as if the entire bone forming "cell team" is receiving instructions comparable to both offensive and defensive football coaches simultaneously talking. At any time, the bone can show excessive resorption or, paradoxically, too much bone is being formed. Both stages can co-exist at the same time. However, the bone formation is very abnormal and structurally weak, leading to bone pain and deformity. Finally, a stage is entered where the bone activity stops, a burned-out phase. Here bone pain lessens, but the weak bone is subject to fracturing.

In Paget's disease, calcium and phosphorous measurements in the blood and urine are normal, but other tests are available to determine the stage and extent of disease. Bone alkaline phosphatase measurement in the blood can often be very elevated indicating the bone formation stage. If very elevated, this is sufficient to begin treating the disease to prevent fractures. The skull, long bones, spine and pelvis are most frequently involved, and x-rays of these areas are quite striking. The second stage of bone resorption is noted by increased products of collagen breakdown, measured in blood and urine.

As a result of bone deformity in Paget's disease and abnormal growth, several health problems can emerge. Enlargement of the skull can lead to hearing loss, headache, ringing in the ears or dizziness. Compression of spinal cord nerves from Paget's disease of the base of the skull or the spine, can produce symptoms of a stroke. Increased blood supply to the rapidly growing bone causes warmth at the site of involved bones. Rarely, this disease can produce a form of heart failure due to demands on the heart to provide enough blood for the bones.

Treatment

Treatment of Paget's disease has two goals. The first is to relieve the bone pain, and the second is to prevent or arrest the complications noted above, including fracture. One treatment used to inhibit Osteoclast resorption of bone is the hormone Calcitonin. This treatment limits the degree of bone impairment and fracture. Injected Calcitonin is also effective in lessening the pain, often within several weeks of starting the medication.

More recently, bisphosphonates such as Alendronate (Fosamax) that are used for Osteoporosis are frequently given orally but in much higher amounts; four times the level of what is used in Osteoporosis. Bisphosphonates are quite effective for the treatment of Paget's Disease. In advanced cases, combination therapy of several drugs can be used.

Inherited Diseases of the Bone and Connective Tissue

Bone disease may show up as early as the first year of life. A rare disease of bone that is seen at birth, Osteogenesis Imperfecta (that means imperfect bone formation). This is due to a defect in the collagen backbone of bone. Individuals with this disease often have deformed arms and legs. They may have difficulty in expanding their chests when they breathe which can lead to Pneumonia. Other also may develop abnormal retinas in the eyes and deafness. This disease can cause aortic aneurysms (weakening and ballooning of the aortic artery that can rupture). This occurs because the elastic lining of the large blood vessels are also abnormal. Those suffering from this disorder often do not live beyond age 10.

A less severe, yet deforming abnormality of bone formation, is Achondroplastic Dwarfing. This most common form of dwarfing is not the result of an abnormality of growth hormone, but rather of bone formation. The munchkins who pointed Judy Garland to help her make her way on the yellow brick road to the Land of Oz, are the most remembered examples of this disease. The disease results in both arms and legs being disproportionately short: the circus sideshow dwarf is usually afflicted with this disease. More subtle abnormalities of elastic tissue, cartilage, or bone formation are seen in individuals who bruise easily, or those who have "double-jointedness". An example of such severely affected individuals is the "Indian-Rubber Man". He can tie his body into knots.

Another example of elastic tissue disease is seen in long, spindly people with huge arm spans and spider-like fingers. These individuals often die of unsuspected, burst aortic aneurysms or heart failure and suffer from Marfan's syndrome (Abraham Lincoln was believed to be affected by this disease). This disease has recently been found to result from a mutation of the gene which leads to the production of the protein elastin. The resulting abnormal elastin protein is a major part of elastic fibers, that are therefore defective and prone to rupture.

Overview

Sensitive new tools of scientific investigation allow us to understand the defects of protein production or action that contribute to bone disease development. Similarly, even some birth bone disorders are potentially treatable. Investigation of whether key genes are normal led us to abnormal genes and therefore proteins responsible for these diseases. Understanding the roles of collagen production, calcium incorporation and the regulation of the functions of the osteoblast and osteoclast by other hormones has led to new treatment strategies. On the horizon, replacement of abnormal genes with normal genes (gene therapy) to prevent or cure some of these disorders is feasible although not yet available. Such therapy raises important ethical issues. Our society must develop guidelines to ensure that people suffering with these diseases can be treated without delay to gain greatly improved quality and quantity of life.

Menopause

General Aspects

I n North America, menopause often occurs in women who enter their 50s. Obviously, earlier removal of the ovaries with or without uterine hysterectomy brings on a surgical menopause. Menopause results mainly from the loss of estrogen production in the ovary. There often is a variety of symptoms that occur upon menopause. Hot flashes with night (and daytime) sweating is common. Mood changes include irritability and anger. Abnormal sleep patterns contribute to memory decrease, and feelings of unclear thinking can occur. Sometimes the symptoms are due to anxiety and depression that may have started before menopause, now made stronger. Many of these symptoms are often improved by reducing stress, weight loss if overweight, and focusing on what one enjoys.

Over the counter medications and foods such as soy that activates the estrogen receptor are not predictable to help reduce menopausal symptoms. Hormone replacement therapy or other medications that will be discussed can be used to minimize many of the symptoms. Organs are less able to carry out their functions. Impaired normal function of the urinary bladder and vagina can occur especially in the absence of estrogen. Loss of vaginal strength can lead to painful intercourse.

Hormone Replacement

In women who have not undergone uterus and ovary surgical removal but developed menopause with aging, estrogen plus progesterone is prescribed in low concentrations. This can be done by oral pills taken continuously. Alternatively, estrogen patches and oral progesterone (micronized is the preferred form of the drug) can be used. Together they reduce the risk of some consequences when estrogen alone is taken by pills. Using estrogen patches results in a reduced likelihood of developing leg vein thrombosis (blood clots) and possible thrombus-embolus into the lungs. This occurs much more commonly in obese women. Blood clots used to occur more often when contraceptive pills containing high amounts of estrogen and progesterone were used in the 1960 and 1970s. Also, adding smoking cigarettes to taking estrogen and progesterone pills increases the likelihood that a venous thrombosis occurs, and smoking should be avoided.

The pills of micronized progesterone are better than earlier formulations. Progesterone reduces the ability of estrogen to stimulate uterine cancer, to less than 1% risk. A concern that is based upon the Woman's Health Initiative (WHI) results, where 25,000 women were enrolled to receive either hormone replacement or placebo (no hormone). The key reason for this study is to determine what is the incidence of breast cancer. Post-menopausal women taking a placebo had an 11 % development of breast cancer, where the women taking a combination of estrogen and progesterone raised this to approximately 14/100 women (14%). However, 86% of the latter women did not develop breast cancer and there are many positive effects of estrogen in older women. Women who have had a hysterectomy and ovaries removed, may _take estrogen alone_. The incidence of breast cancer in women taking estrogen alone was slightly _reduced_ compared to_the placebo group. This means that it is only when both sex hormones are taken together is there an increase in breast cancer. There is also some evidence that women taking hormone replacement at age 65-70 develop a *slightly* higher incidence of heart infarction (heart attack) but this was only when estrogen was started late in life. There is data from the WHI clinical trial that estrogen can prevent heart attacks when started at early menopause (33% reduction in heart attacks compared to women taking placebo).

Another form of hormone replacement, rather than patches and progesterone pills is a drug called Duavee. This is a combination of ethinyl estradiol (estrogen) and a SERM, bazedoxifene. The latter is like raloxifene or tamoxifen. Bazedoxifene blocks the effects of estrogen in the breast and uterus, thus preventing additional cancers that occur from estrogen alone (uterus) or estrogen plus progesterone replacement (breast). Duavee has been approved in the USA by the FDA for treating post-menopausal symptoms and preventing osteoporosis.

If women either do not want or it is advisable to not take estrogen, non-hormone therapy can be used. Although some menopausal symptoms like "hot flashes" can be reduced, many other positive effects of estrogen include preventing osteoporosis is not aided by alternative post-menopausal drugs described below. Most often drugs that reduce post-menopausal symptoms are serotonin reuptake or serotonin and norepinephrine reuptake inhibitors (SSRI or SNRI drugs). Low dose of *paroxetine mesylate* is the FDA approved, non-hormone drug for reducing severity of hot flashes. A second drug, gabapentin reduces many symptoms that may be worse at night (sleep disorder, anxiety, other symptoms of menopause). For avoiding pain on sexual relations, vaginal creams and moisturizers are helpful. Vaginal estrogen cream at a low dose can be used as it is not absorbed into the blood but acts only locally for symptom relief.

Positive effects of estrogen replacement after menopause

In the first few years after menopause the lack of estrogen correlates to increased visceral (often abdominal) fat gain of 6-8 pounds. This occurs because estrogen limits the development of fat from stem cells. Estrogen also stimulates energy expenditure by increasing brown fat-stimulated heat production that burns calories often stored in fat. Estrogen also limits appetite and stimulates physical activity. These effects are the result of estrogen action especially in a portion of the brain, the hypothalamus gland.

Gain of weight contributes to decreased normal action of insulin, that can contribute to the development of Diabetes Mellitus. This is especially problematic in overweight, poorly active women. Unrelated to the weight loss, estrogen also acts to enhance the action of insulin. As mentioned, estrogen prevents osteoporosis in post-menopausal women.

Estrogen loss also may promote diseases of the brain. Men have 50% more Parkinson's disease than woman, even though this disease is most often seen in aged individuals. There is both human and animal models that show estrogen can reduce severe symptoms and prevent the development of the disease. The latter is possibly caused by preserving the brain neuron cells that secrete dopamine, a neurotransmitter (chemical) that is crucial to normal walking and overall activity. More research as to the mechanisms is required.

There is conflicting data about estrogen and stroke. In the Woman's Health Initiative clinical trial, estrogen was usually started many years after the menopause in older women and caused a small increase in the occurrence of stroke. However both animal studies and some studies in woman, show that *early* use of estrogen just as the menopause is emerging indicates this sex hormone can prevent stroke. In mice studies, estrogen given at the time of an induced stroke strongly limits the amount of brain damage. More studies in humans are important. There is some evidence that starting estrogen early in menopause decreases the development of Alzheimers Disease. Based upon animal models, experiments suggest many other important effects of estrogen occur through binding receptors in many parts of the brain.

Menopause in men

There is no agreed upon evidence that men undergo something equivalent to menopause. With aging, testosterone levels often gradually decrease in older men. This can cause a loss of libido (sex drive) and have a small effect on the ability to have an erection. The latter is more often due to the loss of blood flow to the penis, resulting from loss of nitric oxide. This occurs in many arteries in the body with aging. Drugs such as Viagra stimulate nitric oxide formation to enhance erections. Other complaints that are common with older men are loss of strength and increased fatigue. Some studies suggest testosterone replacement (patch or injection) enhances libido and strength and stamina. However loss of strength and stamina are not clearly proved to occur because of low testosterone.

It is important when giving testosterone to men that monitoring blood tests for possible over-stimulation of blood red cell formation. There is a concern that high red blood cell numbers can lead to thrombosis and stroke, Interestingly, in all men, testosterone is converted to estrogen. The estrogen is quite important to men's health, including limiting abdominal fat, decreasing accelerated atherosclerosis, reducing unfavorable cholesterol (LDL cholesterol) and increasing favorable cholesterol (HDL cholesterol), and enhancing normal insulin action. In older men, the estrogen generated from testosterone is responsible for 75% of limiting the development of Osteoporosis. So, as I often state when giving a lecture on this, the men in the audience need to pay attention to their "feminine side" (just kidding).

Gene Therapy

The sunlight glinted into the hospital room, announcing the beginning of Steven Arn's journey. Today, he would have definitive treatment for the disease which had made his life unbearable for two years: He was to now receive gene therapy. The chemotherapy which had been used as traditional treatment for his leukemia was discovered many years ago. Instead, inserting "Designer Genes" into the cells from his body, as the doctors had called them, is the state of the art for some diseases. Here a normal gene is produced and inserted into his white blood cells, the lymphocytes. The cells are then returned to Steven's body so that the lymphocytes reproduce and destroy the cancer cells.

Also, the protein products of these genes stimulate the body to produce additional proteins which kill the leukemic cells by stimulating his impaired immune system. This is known as Cart-T therapy. The doctors were practicing a form of molecular tinker toys, redesigning the DNA of his cells to cure the cancer which had ravaged Steven's body and spirit. This is the state of emerging medical treatment for increasing numbers of diseases.

This seemingly fictional account is occurring as you read this. Gene therapy is a reality. Several diseases are first routinely *identified* by gene DNA technologies. New genetic tests to establish the diseases of Muscular

Dystrophy, Cystic Fibrosis, and Marfan's Syndrome are available for general screening purposes. Molecular techniques allow the screening and the identification of individuals with Huntington's Disease, Amyotrophic Lateral Sclerosis, (Lou Gehrig's Diseases), and Neurofibromatosis. Abnormal genes and the resulting altered proteins that drive various cancers then provide treatment targets. As a result, medical therapies have greatly improved.

Recently, gene replacement of a mutated gene with the normal gene, making the normal protein named transthyretin has shown great ability to resolve the symptoms that men with *Primary Amyloidosis* endure (rare disease).

Some women weigh the burden of whether they want to know if they have abnormal BRCA 1 or 2 genes that run in their family. The mutant (not normal) BRCA genes predispose most of these women to breast or ovarian cancer development. *What should they do with this information?* Some women elect to have their ovaries and breasts surgically removed.

Eventually the family doctor's office will begin to resemble a gene research laboratory, because common diseases will be identified at early stages of development by gene profile. Diagnosis of disease will be as routine as determining a red blood cell count currently. Many diseases are the result of a single mutation (abnormality) of a single gene and will be identified. This provides the basis for preventive medical practice and/or informed counselling. Although still early in the use of gene replacement, this area continues to grow. This leads to normal protein function and will be the permanent remedy for many diseases in the future.

Identification of the gene or genes responsible for a specific disease first requires locating the important gene among millions of pieces of DNA in humans. The first attempts were like finding the needle in the haystack. However, refinements of screening procedures have accelerated the pace by which we can find the culprits causing a specific disease. The next step is to understand what proteins result from gene expression. This is crucial because therapy will follow only after we understand the *function of the protein products.*

For instance, the normal gene which is altered in cystic fibrosis (**CF**) codes for a protein which sits in the outer layer of many cells. The CF protein directs chloride and sodium in and out of the cell. In fact, children suffering this disease from birth excessively excrete chloride and sodium. New treatment with a drug called Trikafta has recently been shown as very useful in individuals with mutation of the key gene causing this disease. Interestingly, young girls undergoing puberty develop a severe increase of this disease due to estrogen action.

In CF, disorders of the intestine and bile drainage are common, and males are almost always infertile. These individuals develop severe lung disease, and pancreas disease leading to malnutrition and poor growth. Also they often develop urinary tract abnormal function. Future therapy will be directed toward inserting a normal gene, resulting in a normal protein inserted into the cell. This will then allow the regulated passage of chloride and sodium in a normal fashion in and out of cells. This can cure the disease. Gene therapy is now used to treat Sickle Cell Anemia, Thalassemia, and diseases of the immune system due to a single abnormal gene.

There are children who have abnormalities of the growth hormone gene and resulting protein that is made in the pituitary gland. They are very short as a result. This could conceivably be treated with gene therapy in the future. Of course safety is established first. The diagnosis and treatment of diseases will increasingly occur through genetic techniques. This may be applied to forms of male and female infertility, often affecting hormone production. Determining the entire human genome (all genes) has advanced genetic approaches for diagnosis and treatment of disease. Soon, everyone will have their genes determined. This will be done to identify abnormal genes that promote development of diseases in the person's future. This allows early prevention or treatment.

Crisper-Cas9 editing removes abnormal genes that cause disease, and this technique is now being tested for human disease application. A very recent example as mentioned above is in the treatment of a disease called Amyloidosis. Six patients underwent Crisper-Cas gene editing resulting in very reduced disease symptoms.

As gene-replacement techniques progress, many moral and ethical issues will be raised. For instance, should genetic information be sought about a non-lethal disease? The parents to be may decide to embrace abortion of the fetus. As our society wrestles with questions that polarize neighbors, friends and family members, the dilemmas raised by application of genetic techniques will cause more debate about abortion. This is not meant to cause anti-scientific waves of protest, or a desire to return to 19th century medical practice. Rather, discussion will stimulate concerned people to anticipate, debate, and enact guidelines which will also serve as a blueprint for the future efforts of biological scientists. Only with the consent of society will the pace of scientific discovery match its potential.

Hormones and Cancer

Many hormones contribute to the growth of numerous tumors. However only a few *cause* a tumor. As an example, high insulin levels in the blood promotes the development of breast cancer, especially if the woman is obese and her glucose is not well controlled. The tumor uses the excessive glucose and insulin for fuel and growth of the cancer. Similarly, colon cancer is promoted in this way.

Sex hormones, Estrogen and Progesterone, cause 75% of all breast cancers in women. Less than 20% of breast cancers don't express the protein receptors for these steroid hormones. In these individuals, *no direct causation* by the steroid hormones occurs. Estrogen *alone* with no progesterone does not seem to cause breast cancer. Woman who had a hysterectomy and ovaries removed may take estrogen alone for symptoms of menopause. These women do not have an increased rate of developing breast cancer. The was shown in the Woman's Health Initiative clinical trial, involving 25,000 women either taking Estrogen, or Estrogen plus Progesterone (if the uterus is intact), or placebo. Women take the Progesterone to protect the uterus from the effects of Estrogen that by itself induces growth and development of a tumor in the lining of the uterus.

However, Estrogen strongly promotes the expression of the Progesterone receptor in breast cells. The two hormones together are very important for the initial and later stages of development of most of breast tumors. In addition to any surgery or radiation prescribed by an Oncologist, additional treatment occurs with a drug that blocks Estrogen production. Importantly it is necessary to block especially the sex steroid made in the breast. Inhibition of Estrogen production results from taking aromatase inhibitor medication, like letrozole or anastrazole, These drugs are very often used in women with this malignancy. Additionally, to further lower the effects of Estrogen, drugs like fulvestrant block estrogen action at its receptor. Some tumors progress, fueled by the action of other growth factors, These tumors often lose the expression of Estrogen and Progesterone receptors, and often show metastases to other sites in the body (brain, bone, lung). Estrogen also stimulates some forms of cancer in the ovaries. But interestingly this sex steroid inhibits liver cancer development. The ratio of men to woman who develop liver malignancy is often due to chronic virus hepatitis. The male to female ratio is as much as 7 to 1. The difference between men and women is in part because Estrogen blocks the inflammation from Hepatitis B infection in the liver that can progress to liver failure and cancer.

The main sex steroid in men, Testosterone, does not seem to cause but does *strongly promote the growth* of early and later stages of prostate cancer. Importantly, the treatment of this malignancy is surgery and/or radiation to the prostate. But often the production of Testosterone from the testicles is blocked with medication. Also, the Testosterone receptor function is blocked or the receptor is degraded by drugs that are specific for the Androgen (Testosterone) receptor.

Interestingly, *mutations* of the Estrogen receptor (where the DNA has been changed from normal) in women with breast cancer and the Androgen receptor in men with prostate cancer allow the tumors to grow and develop even in almost the complete absence of the sex steroid. This is a very important cause of tumors that no longer respond to the usual medicine therapies. Therefore, the current focus in these malignancies is to find new <u>drugs that degrade the receptors</u> and therefore prevent tumor progression.

Conclusion

There are many examples in this book where too little hormone produces disease such as when Insulin decreases, Diabetes results. Or, too much hormone, as with parathyroid hormone, causes high calcium and promotes Osteoporosis. The key to a healthy body is to maintain normal amounts and activities of the many hormones secreted by almost every organ in the body. Measuring hormones by your health care practitioner will define potential problems early, to prevent many symptoms that often occur.